YOGA ZONE

yoga
for
life

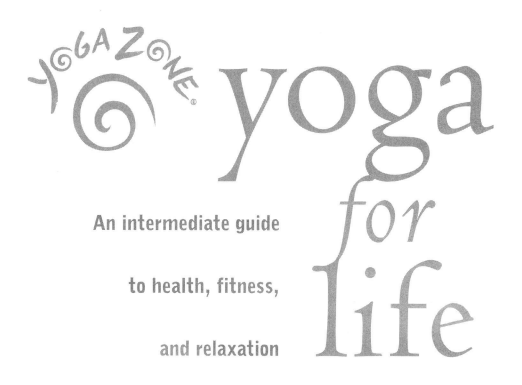

yoga for life

An intermediate guide

to health, fitness,

and relaxation

YOGA MASTER ALAN FINGER

with AL BINGHAM and ELIZABETH ROYLES PARKER

THREE RIVERS PRESS • NEW YORK

Published by Three Rivers Press, New York, New York.
Member of the Crown Publishing Group, a division of Random House, Inc.
www.crownpublishing.com

THREE RIVERS PRESS and the tugboat design are registered trademarks
of Random House, Inc.

Printed in the United States of America

Design by Maggie Hinders

Library of Congress Cataloging-in-Publication Data
Finger, Alan, 1946–
Yoga Zone yoga for life: an intermediate guide to health, fitness, and relaxation / Alan
Finger, with Al Bingham.—1st ed.
I. Yoga—Popular works. I. Bingham, Al. II. Title.
RA781.7 .F563 2004
613.7'046—dc22   2003015477

ISBN 0-609-80406-5

10 9 8 7 6 5 4 3 2 I

First Edition

To my teacher and my father, Kavi Yogiraj Mani Finger,

who took maha samadhi in July 2001.

His passion, enthusiasm, and humor are still alive in me.

ॐ

CONTENTS

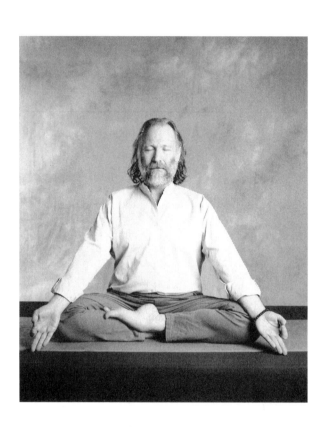

A LIFE'S JOURNEY

DEAR READER,

IT IS MY SINCERE HOPE that you will use some of the practices in *Yoga for Life* to navigate a path through this sometimes stressful and confusing world. Yoga can be a valuable way to combat stress and discover things about yourself and your place in this world that you may never have dreamed possible. Yoga, when you embrace it as an integral part of your life, can provide an internal compass that will lead you on a wholly realized, fulfilled, beautiful journey.

As you go off into the world, taking your yoga practice with you, remind yourself that at any given moment you are exactly where you need to be. Instead of accepting what is right in front of us, we sometimes succumb to hyperactive energy and make abrupt changes before we truly understand a situation. One of our most deeply ingrained societal myths tells us that extreme satisfaction is to be found in making drastic life changes. In the movies, larger-than-life characters quit their jobs, divorce their spouses, get fantastic makeovers, and drive off into the sunset with wittier, more spontaneous love interests. A more realistic sequel—but one that would probably never make it to the big screen—would feature a hero facing the same internal issues that were present before the drastic life change took place.

You do not have to completely overhaul who you are, what you are doing, and where your life is heading to find fulfillment in life. The truth is, if you make simple, directed changes, everything else will follow in course. Shifting your internal compass slightly makes all the difference: when a mariner changes his course by a few degrees, it can mean the difference between ending up in North America or South America. Instead of taking drastic action, we need to be consistent in our actions, and that sets us on a purposeful, gradual path to enlightenment.

Surprisingly, acting consistently is much harder than acting radically. It requires significant discipline and effort. The good news, though, is that consistent mindfulness can completely transform your life, not to mention the lives of those around you. No matter what course you take, you will encounter challenges and difficulty. Your internal compass, however, will help you navigate through whatever comes your way. If you tried to steer a submarine by looking out a window, you wouldn't be able to see very far ahead of you—as soon as you encountered a school of fish, you might become disoriented and steer off course. But if the onboard navigational instruments were guiding you, then when that school of fish came along, you would watch it out the window and marvel at its beauty.

Simple internal changes may have dramatic consequences. Tiny drops of water can wear a hole through the hardest granite. You may end up changing jobs, switching careers, adopting a different lifestyle, or finding a different partner, but you will be awake to the process. It will be a purpose-driven journey rather than one born of a knee-jerk reaction.

When you are being motivated by your soul's voice, you are tuned in to the omnipresence of divine intelligence and aid. The law of karma makes sure that we never miss the lessons we are due to get; we will always get a second, third, or fourth opportunity—however many it takes—to learn the lessons that we need.

Your soul is there. You cannot help but find it if you keep looking. It is not something your mind can wrap itself around; you cannot think your way to it, you must act in order to experience it. You might discover your soul in an instant or after years of looking. In the big picture time is of no importance. Maintain your curiosity, and you will be astounded and mystified by what you come across.

Life will continue to happen to you. You can merely return over and over again to practice. The *Yoga Sutras* remind us that if our practice is consistent over a long time, we will find our heart's desire. Do not expect overnight changes. Do not expect a rosy, blissful existence. Instead, use whatever situations come your way as opportunities for growth, and then you will truly know, moment to moment, that everything is indeed as it should be.

With warmest wishes for your journey,

Hari om,

ALAN FINGER

YOGA ZONE

yoga
for
life

1

YOGA FOR LIFE

*The practice of yoga is the commitment to become established
in the state of freedom.*

PATANJALI, *YOGA SUTRAS*, CHAPTER 1, VERSE 13

THE BLISS OF HAVING JUST FINISHED A SUCCESSFUL YOGA PRACTICE IS UNLIKE ANYTHING ELSE IN THE WORLD. AN HOUR OF MAINTAINING FOCUSED CONTROL OVER THE BODY, BREATH, AND MIND REENERGIZES YOU, NO MATTER HOW tired, stressed, or uninterested you felt at the start. Serene energy unfolds, and you feel balanced, powerful, strong, refreshed, calm, and at peace. Indeed, after their very first yoga class, many beginning students stand a little straighter, feel a little stronger, breathe a little more mindfully, and enjoy life with a pleasant new combination of ease and awareness. They experience the sensation of release and well-being that comes after they have explored the core of their body, stretched their muscles, and focused on their breath. It is a captivating feeling! It is only natural to seek to expand this harmony beyond the practice mat and into your daily activities, and that is the idea behind *Yoga Zone Yoga for Life.*

There is no mystical explanation for why practicing yoga makes people feel so good—the answer is purely scientific. The Sanskrit term *samadhi* refers to the blissful feeling that one experiences at the end of practice and that has been sought for thousands of years. When you do the poses and breathing exercises, and when you gain focus over your thoughts and your body, you achieve rhythms in your brain that you cannot achieve in the course of normal life. First, your brain waves enter an alpha rhythm similar to that of beginning sleep, and then when you become more and more practiced, you can enter into the delta rhythms of deep sleep—all while remaining fully awake.

In fact, at the Menninger Foundation in Kansas, Dr. Elmer Green observed an advanced yogi, Swami Rama, practice a self-induced state of deep relaxation called *yoga nidra,* also known as "the sleepless sleep." Swami Rama was able to lower himself through deeper and deeper states of unconsciousness, while simultaneously maintaining an aural awareness of all that was occurring around him in the laboratory setting. By monitoring the yogi's brain waves, Dr. Green confirmed that they were becoming slower and slower. Swami Rama moved progressively toward a near-hibernation state, and his senses disengaged in turn—first smell, then taste, sight, and touch, and finally, the sense of hearing, which explains why he was still able to hear what was happening in the room.

You are probably familiar with a similar mental state even if you don't think you are. Your brain usually enters this so-called "hypnogogic" condition, albeit only for a few seconds or at most a few minutes, as your body drifts off to sleep. During meditation you are able to induce and extend that mental state between consciousness and sleep, or *yoga nidra.*

When you achieve control over your brain rhythms, remarkable results may begin to take place in your life. You will feel more in control of your emotions and your responses to the world because you will be more cognizant of the difference between reality and fleeting emotion. Small, miraculous occurrences may happen: you will be thinking of someone, and your phone will ring—that person is calling you; you will dream of something, and it will happen the next day; your golf or tennis swing will attain that once-in-a-blue-moon effortless perfection. These sorts of miraculous occurrences—or in Sanskrit, *siddhis*—make you feel that you have a connection, albeit brief, to some larger universal force.

According to the tenets of yoga, a *siddhi* occurs when you are able to channel the intelligence from the universe into your daily life. Essentially this means that with meditation, physical postures, and control of the breath, you can become aware of magic in your life. Indeed, the wonder and splendor of the universe is well within your grasp, as it has been for millions of yoga practitioners over thousands of years.

Not only can yoga create magic in your life, it can also provide a framework for seeing and understanding the true nature of things, for distinguishing between what is real and what is illusory. Paramahansa Yogananda, an eminent yoga teacher who initiated my father into yoga practice, used a compelling analogy to illustrate how easy it is to lose sight of reality. When we go to the movies, Yogananda said, we forget that what we are really doing is staring at a white wall. What is projected onto that wall is so captivating that we become distracted in laughing or crying, in feeling scared, confused, or amazed. We forget the blank white screen that is really there underneath it all. How can we possibly forget something so obvious? Easily—our minds are not focused.

In the state of yoga, we experience that pure background consciousness (the white wall) that exists behind the moving reality of our lives (the projected images). It is only when we are experiencing the pure background of the universe that duality no longer exists. We are in a state of oneness. Only in that ultimate state of union, a union with all things, is the mind no longer distracted. This may help you understand why *yoga*, a Sanskrit word with many layers of meaning, can be translated as "union," "oneness," and "yoking" simultaneously.

The practice of yoga helps transition us from the stressful dual world to the underlying stress-free reality of oneness. Because we must exist in a dual world as we conduct our daily lives, yoga also teaches us how to find as much balance and harmony as possible.

An Ancient Tradition

AS YOU BECOME AWARE of the scope of the yoga tradition and the possibilities that lie just beyond your daily practice mat, you will understand more clearly why yoga has been enchanting its practitioners for thousands of years. Present-day yoga derives from roots that are millennia old: Patanjali's *Yoga Sutras*, written two thousand years ago, remains the original how-to book on yoga, and many people are surprised and awed to learn that the postures, or *asanas*, practiced today were originally developed in India more than five thousand years ago. Nevertheless the primarily physical yoga practiced in the West today is just a small part of an ancient discipline. Yoga did not emerge five thousand years ago in response to a need for a more holistic way of exercising. Indeed, millenniums ago people did not need "the workout" that we crave today. But as time has marched on, so too has awareness that these teachings can be applied equally to life's grand mysteries—questions like "Who am I?" and "Why am I here?"—as well as to less metaphysical questions such as "Why can't I bend over and touch my toes anymore?" In the following pages we will explore both kinds of questions, and the long tradition of asking them.

Any bookstore or library will present you with a trove of books about yoga, written both by ancient sages and by present-day yogis. The vastness of yoga studies can be intimidating to the eager student looking to advance and expand his or her yoga practice. Yoga practice has many levels, and beginning yoga students seek answers to many different questions: How can yoga aid in my recovery from illness, injury, or stress? How does mental stress manifest itself in my body? How can I locate and work out tension in my neck, pelvis, or legs? How do breathing exercises, called *pranayama,* connect with the *asanas?* Is it really yoga if I am just working on my breath?

On a different level, you may now be wondering how yoga can create, through *samadhi* and *siddhis,* magic in your life. How can yoga help you find your purpose in the world and a feeling of oneness with the universe? How do the *Yoga Sutras* written by Patanjali connect to the physical postures? *Yoga Zone Yoga for Life* will meet your study of yoga where you are today and offer some valuable guidance on how to focus and deepen your practice so that you can feel its maximum benefits wherever you need them.

ISHTA Yoga

THE STYLE OF YOGA taught in the Yoga Zone videotapes and books is called ISHTA yoga. ISHTA is an acronym for the Integrated Sciences of Hatha, Tantra, and Ayurveda, but *ishta* is also a Sanskrit word that means "individual" or "personalized." That double meaning is significant because one of yoga's major strengths is its ability to be tailored to an individual's needs. In this book you will learn how to use focused, specific yoga practices to address problems and questions you may have in your life.

Hatha yoga is the basis of many different schools of yoga; it involves the simultaneous practice of physical postures and steady, deep breathing. In some schools of yoga, such as Iyengar yoga, hatha poses are held for long periods of time, bringing the focus to realignment and strengthening of the body. In other styles of yoga, *asana* positions and steady breathing are connected in continuously flowing sequences called *vinyasas,* which are more vigorous and fast-paced. Yoga Zone's ISHTA yoga uses postures in both ways, depending on the student's individual needs. Another hallmark of ISHTA yoga is the constant, careful attention paid to the breath, no matter how quickly or slowly the poses are entered.

My father, Mani Finger, and I originally developed the ISHTA yoga style in South Africa, based on the teachings of various master yoga teachers who stayed with us in our home or whom my father met during his travels. Among those who contributed significant inspiration to this new style were Paramahansa Yogananda, Yogananda's brother Vishnu Ghosh, Swami Sivananda, Swami Venkatesananda, Swami Nishraisananda, and the Tantric master Shuddhanand Bharati.

When I moved to the United States in the 1970s, I founded the Yoga Zone studios, and since then I have worked with my Yoga Zone teachers to modify and expand ISHTA yoga so that it can accommodate the needs of those who are drawn to practice it.

You have probably picked up *Yoga Zone Yoga for Life* because you wish to expand your yoga practice, and if so, you have come to the right place. Many students, familiar with the basic *asanas* and tenets of yoga, wish to delve into their practice with more rigor but are uncertain how best to proceed. Beginners often assume that the goal of yoga is to assume difficult postures effortlessly and with utmost flexibility. This is not the case. Yoga's goal is not to tie your body into a pretzel! Becoming truly advanced in yoga practice is not just a matter of gaining increased flexibility and balance, although those things are byproducts of a rigorous practice. Rather, it necessitates developing a deepened awareness of the body, mind, breath, and the world around us. Attaining this awareness is much more difficult than the most challenging *asana,* but it is truly rewarding.

2

REDUCING STRESS

Distractions make the body restless, the breathing coarse, and the mind agitated. They result in suffering. But they can be eliminated if the mind is brought to a single focus.

PATANJALI, *YOGA SUTRAS*, CHAPTER I, VERSES 31–32

EVERYONE EXPERIENCES STRESS—IT IS A PHENOMENON AS OLD AS THE HUMAN RACE. THE FAST PACE OF TWENTY-FIRST-CENTURY LIFE PROVOKES THE STRESS RESPONSE—AND EXACERBATES ITS NEGATIVE SIDE EFFECTS—probably more than any other time in history. Never before have people experienced so many pressures in the course of a single day: pressures to earn money, be successful in a career or job, meet deadlines and goals, pay bills, drive the right car, wear the right clothes, live in a nice home, and even more important, raise healthy, well-adjusted children and be a generous and considerate friend, colleague, spouse, and family member.

If these pressures and responsibilities have not affected you physically and emotionally, you are lucky. Most people, however, are physically and emotionally overwrought by daily stress. You may feel that there is not enough time in the day to fulfill all your countless responsibilities. You may feel that you have let down your family or friends in some way. You may have gotten yourself into some sticky situation and are having some trouble extricating yourself. You feel as if you are the only one who has ever suffered from these problems. In fact, all of these emotions are common, but knowing that others feel the same way does not make them any more bearable to someone suffering from stress.

In today's society it is common, unfortunately, to get trapped in a cycle of stress. The original biological reason for developing the stress response was survival. The fight-or-flight response provided early human beings with the physical means to escape danger: the sympathetic nervous system kicks into high gear; the heart rate speeds up, increasing blood flow to the arms and legs by 300 percent; energy diverts away from digestion; adrenaline pumps through the blood; the pupils dilate, decreasing peripheral vision; and the breath becomes shallower and more rapid.

When the stressful situation disappears, nature intends for the body to return to a balanced state. Unfortunately, in this fast-paced culture nature backfires, and we often get stuck in the fight-or-flight mode. Before we have recovered and rebalanced from the last stressful event, the next challenge is already upon us. Stress becomes chronic and overrides the relaxation response; the body loses its chance to recover. As subsequent stressors appear, we are less and less capable of dealing with them. Often people resort to alcohol, cigarettes, binge eating, and other coping mechanisms to deal with the stress, causing even more harm to themselves.

Exploring and Releasing Stress with Yoga

IF LEFT UNCHECKED and unexamined, stress can take physical root in your body. The large muscles in your legs, the quadriceps and hamstrings, may become tense and inflexible. Can you relax them completely? Probably not. You may also carry tension in the muscles of your neck, back, pelvis, jaw, or some other area. The tension may be so normal that you do not even notice it anymore, but that does not mean it is not harmful. Similarly, emotional stress can become such a natural state that you no longer notice that you are sleeping poorly, overreacting to small problems, or cultivating an outlook of doom and gloom. Worse, over a long period of time, physical and emotional stress can cause many physical ailments: high blood pressure, heart disease, migraine headaches, back trouble . . . the list, unfortunately, continues.

Clearly, it would do you good to find a way to release yourself from this vicious circle! If you are like most people, however, you are accustomed to feeling uncomfortable, and you cannot begin to remember what true relaxation, stillness, and peace feel like. To recover that peace, you must change your outlook. Certainly this is easier said than done, but unlearning stress, like unlearning any bad habit, is a process that begins with the intention to change. When we are confronted with stress, we can choose either to accept the damage it wreaks on our bodies and emotions or to examine and confront that damage. Removing yourself from the grip of stress is difficult because stressed behavior is so practiced and habitual. But bit by bit, using yoga, you can certainly reverse the pattern. Practice a new vision: learn to greet the onset of stress positively, because it signals a situation that is causing you discomfort, giving you an opportunity to break old, harmful patterns of thought and behavior and consciously create healthier new ones. The key is self-examination.

Most people find the practice of yoga strenuous precisely because it involves constant physical and mental self-examination, along with attention to the breath to bridge the space between the mind and the body. Concentration of this sort is rare and can feel a bit unnatural at first. No other form of exercise is so mindful; not even a professional athlete considers each toe, each finger, each vertebra, each inhalation and each exhalation with complete attention, as a yogi does.

With continued practice, you too can cultivate a strong self-awareness that will help you deal constructively with any stressful situation. Yoga's physical postures will show you the effects that stress has carved into your body, such as those tight calves or inflexible hamstrings to which you have long since grown accustomed. Luckily, *asanas* also give you the means to work out that tension, inflexibility, and soreness, and over the weeks, months, and years when you practice yoga, these symptoms will gradually dissipate. Next, *pranayama,* the study of the breath, will help you develop control over both mind and body, as the increased oxygen flow calms your mind and oxygenates your blood and muscles. Different forms of *pranayama* can help you search variously for control, balance, harmony, stress release, and much more.

Finally, all Yoga Zone classes include meditation practice in order to work up the discipline needed to achieve the balance, unity, and oneness that are the goal of all yoga. Feel free to focus your attention during meditation on whatever you like: the object of meditation may be something physical (the flame of a candle), something subtle (the sound *om*), or something extremely refined (the spaces that exist in the body, or the pause at the end of the breath). No matter what object is the focus of your meditation, distractions will inevitably come up. To the extent that your mind resists the pull of distraction and remains focused on the object, you will come closer to the true experience of yoga. No matter how practiced you are in yoga and meditation, the relaxation that arises will be profoundly healing; for the beginner it approximates a "power nap," and as the laboratory study of Swami Rama in *yoga nidra* shows, the brain waves of practiced meditators can approximate deep sleep. So don't skip the meditation! Contrary to popular belief, the *asana* sequences and *pranayama* are not the main point of yoga; they are simply steps along the way to meditation.

When Stress Gets in the Way of Your Yoga Practice

"I'M TOO STRESSED TO GO TO YOGA CLASS!" Does this sound familiar? You know you are under stress, and maybe you have even identified its source. You have intended to confront your persistent anxiety for a while now. You promised yourself you would practice an *asana* series in the book or a videotaped routine. You make dates to go to yoga classes, but something always seems to get in the way. What can you do?

Patanjali's *Yoga Sutras* identify nine impediments to practicing yoga: illness, dullness, doubts, carelessness, fatigue, inability to resist distractions, erroneous perception, lack of conviction, and instability. Not surprisingly, those same impediments still hinder yoga practitioners today. You need to be aware of the roadblocks that can get in the way of combating the stressful distractions in your life; the same stressors that motivated you to try yoga in the first place may actually prevent you from practicing. So be alert to the obstacles that you come across in the course of your practice. If you know about them in advance, then when they appear, they will not come as a surprise, and you will be prepared to remove them. Read on and see if you can identify a few of your own excuses for not practicing yoga in Patanjali's nine impediments.

ILLNESS

Yoga can always be adapted to the needs of an individual, so if you are sick, your practice need not involve strenuous physical activity or challenging breathing exercises.

There is also a misconception about how long a yoga practice needs to last. When you are not feeling well, you may not want to attend a ninety-minute class that features challenging yoga postures, but spending five minutes at home consciously practicing a few simple poses may be all you need to feel a slight improvement. Listen to your body, and don't push it past its limits. Practicing yoga is not a cure-all; nor is it insurance against the onset of future illness. It can, however, shift your attention away from the illness and help you redefine yourself, so that illness never defines you.

DULLNESS

At times we all feel foggy. Just as literal fog snares rush-hour traffic, a figurative mental "fog" can slow down everything within us. The body is dull, the mind is groggy, the appetite is decreased, and the entire world appears drab and uninspiring.

When you're feeling dull, practicing yoga is a fantastic way to reenergize, if you can find just a little bit of motivation. With yoga, the mind gets sharper, blood starts pumping through the veins, and even the outlook changes. Disbelief and surprise often accompany the moments after someone's first yoga class: "I never knew I could feel this good! Why didn't I start doing this earlier?" No matter how much we hear about yoga, until we experience it ourselves, all that testimony is nothing more than well-intentioned hearsay.

So how then, when you're feeling dreary, can you remind yourself to summon up the energy to practice yoga? Simply put, the best way to overcome dullness is to make an agreement with yourself that wherever you begin is fine. If you start out dull and lethargic, fine. If after three postures you are still feeling dull and lethargic, fine. Just tell yourself to hang in there, because you're on your way—and soon the fog will lift. Yoga's effect is cumulative over time. Slow and steady always reaps the benefits.

DOUBTS

Doubts certainly come up in the course of practicing yoga. You may find yourself asking: What's the point of trying something new at this stage of the game? Am I flexible (strong, focused, balanced, young, athletic, etc.) enough for yoga to work? You may even have doubts about the practice itself; yoga has certainly attracted its share of skeptics. You're wondering: Does yoga work? What good will sitting still and breathing quietly do for me?

Instead of ignoring those doubts, the best way to overcome them is to test them. Scientific studies are under way to investigate the health-related benefits that are so often attributed to the practice of yoga. Already studies have shown that practicing yoga, meditation, or a yoga-derived therapy can be beneficial in healing or managing a wide range of conditions, including hypertension, heart disease, coronary arteriosclerosis (hardening of the arteries), cardiac arrhythmias, high cholesterol, chronic back pain, chronic neck pain, chronic shoulder pain, carpal tunnel syndrome, migraine headaches, bronchial asthma, insomnia, unexplained infertility, premenstrual syndrome, anxiety, mild and moderate depression, anger, fatigue, low self-esteem, a tendency to smoke, drink, or use drugs, eating disorders, work-related stress disorders, stress-related absenteeism, and stress-related declines in worker productivity. Week by week this list lengthens—especially as more and more researchers have discovered yoga themselves. Rather than wait for someone else's opinion, consider yourself a test subject and conduct your own research. Curiosity adds a wonderful element to the yoga practice, so doubt all you want, but keep exploring. Don't take someone else's word for it, no matter how authoritative or knowledgeable they may seem. Instead, tackle those doubts head on and find out the truth for yourself.

CARELESSNESS

Carelessness trips most people up from time to time. When we are lucky, our own carelessness does not have a negative effect on us, but not paying attention to what we are doing frequently produces stress. When we are trying to establish a regular practice of yoga, we can become careless and let other things take priority. The need to complete one last phone call, e-mail, chore, errand, or obligation before we practice yoga can spin us out of control. Suddenly the time we had set aside for yoga has disappeared because now something else *really important* needs to get done.

Carelessness can also extend into the practice itself. Yoga requires us to pay attention to what we are doing, to observe carefully how the mind, body, and breath are interacting. As soon as our attention falters and we start operating on automatic pilot, the practice begins to lose its value. Strive to be attentive in your practice. Focused attention will make you open to inspiration and insight. Physically, you will be able to focus on the messages your body is giving you, avoiding injury and strain. The practice of yoga trains you to become more attentive; over time you will discover that your carelessness diminishes and that you can change some of the habits and patterns that get in the way of thoughtful contemplation.

FATIGUE

Fatigue can be a major roadblock to the practice of yoga. Sometimes, amid the hustle and bustle of the busy modern world, it seems impossible to avoid feeling drained, but with yoga you can restore yourself. The trick is to refuse to let your weariness get in the way and instead let it motivate you. Remember the renewed energy you always feel at the end of practice, and work toward it.

The first step toward overcoming chronic tiredness is to review the pace of your daily schedule. You may simply be on the go a bit too much, and although sometimes a busy schedule is unavoidable, many activities that seem necessary actually are not.

The next time you feel tired, instead of dashing into the local coffee shop for a double espresso, consider resting in place for a few moments. Recognize that your fatigue is sending you a very important message: slow down, your body is not coping well. Yoga can help shift your body out of emergency mode and into a relaxed state that will enable your system to respond appropriately.

In your yoga practice, respect the difference between feelings of laziness and true fatigue. Neither is a reason to forgo any and all practice—there is always something that you can do consciously with your mind, body, and spirit; there is always some practice that can be created. But if you are truly fatigued, make your practice a restful one. Give your body a break.

INABILITY TO RESIST DISTRACTIONS

None of us need a book to tell us that distractions exist and that sometimes people succumb to them. We all know that resisting distractions takes discipline, and that even the best resolve doesn't always work. We know the pint of ice cream in the freezer is a distraction, we have developed strategies to resist it, we know the consequences of not resisting, yet the next thing we know, there we are—pint in hand. As much as our conscious mind may have sworn off that ice cream, the unconscious persists.

The good news is that practicing yoga makes you aware of things you were previously unconscious of, helping to release you from the binds of those harmful habits and motivations. Yoga will not remove the distractions altogether, but luckily, over time your the ability to resist them will become more refined. In the meantime, a good way to resist distractions is to practice dispassion, or *vairagya.* If you are unconcerned about slipping off course, then getting back on course will not be as difficult. The self-deprecating drama that occurs after a slip-up is often more debilitating than the actual wandering. People often criticize themselves internally so much for straying from a diet, for example, that they develop unhealthy obsessions with food—and those obsessions make it harder to resist unhealthy foods the next time. So in your yoga practice, forgive yourself for occasionally being distracted. Recognize that slipping up is part of the learning process, and view your slip-up with dispassion rather than shame. So you fell— okay, then dust yourself off and get back on the mat again.

ERRONEOUS PERCEPTION

Some obstacles that we think are in the way may not actually exist. Conversely, sometimes when all seems smooth sailing ahead, we are misinformed. The approach to erroneous perception is similar to the approach to doubts: test, test, and test again. Blindly accepting something or flat-out rejecting it will never help you, either in life or in yoga. Practicing yoga will refine your ability to perceive clearly, but the senses are limited in their ability to provide us with the complete picture. Keeping an open mind and not jumping to conclusions will serve you well in the practice of yoga.

LACK OF CONVICTION

Lack of conviction keeps many people from continuing with yoga. They are aware of how beneficial the practice is, and they know that continuing to practice will produce additional benefits, but they simply cannot summon up the perseverance to stick with it. Our culture encourages hopping from activity to activity, which makes it even harder to stay resolute. Rather than digging one deep hole, people today often end up digging many shallow holes.

The remedy for this lack of conviction is a familiar one: *vairagya,* or dispassion. Dispassion may seem like an odd prescription for someone who is lacking passion to begin with, but if you tend to be unfocused in your convictions, it makes sense.

Often people who lack the conviction to practice yoga have passions that are focused elsewhere in their pursuits. Having many different convictions or commitments is fine, of course, unless most of your energy is channeled into activities that are not bringing peace and harmony into your life. If work-related stress consumes you, then channeling energy into work-related stress is more important to you than relieving it. Applying a dispassionate approach to that work-related stress will leave you able to increase your passion for the practice of yoga!

INSTABILITY

Having an instability can be a great reason to practice, because, after all, yoga is the science of creating stability. Although instabilities can get in the way of practicing, they need not derail a practice, regardless of whether your instability has its roots in something physical, mental/ emotional, environmental, or chemical. More than anything else, instabilities need to be acknowledged. If, for instance, I fail to acknowledge that I feel unstable bending forward, then I may put excessive pressure on my lower back. If I instead recognize that instability, I can take corrective actions, like bending my knees or starting the motion from a seated position before I attempt it from a standing position.

All nine of the impediments that Patanjali identified may be present simultaneously, or they may take turns showing up in your yoga or life journey. But as we've seen, identifying them and reacting to them with reasoned action is the best way to deal with them. And the more you can accept the inevitability of obstacles, the more you can turn them into opportunities for making positive changes in your life.

Yoga Anywhere

IF YOU ARE IN THE OFFICE and feel a twinge of stress—only an hour left before your presentation, and you haven't written a word!—it is usually not practical or possible to pull out a yoga mat and begin working through some *asana.* Ditto for the stress that comes when you are running late and the train refuses to arrive, or when you are stuck in an interminable line at the movie theater, or when a blind date stands you up at a restaurant. Traditional yoga is not going to work in these situations, but there are some discreet yoga-based exercises that you can do to relieve passing stress and make yourself more comfortable and productive. You will probably even finish writing that presentation because your heart rate will return to normal, your palms will cease sweating, and your mind will be more at ease.

Turn away from your desk so that there is space in front of you. With your feet square on the floor, sit up tall in your chair, imagining that there is a string extending from the top of your head to the ceiling. If you were a marionette, someone could pull you to your feet using the string. Interlace your fingers so that your palms turn out, and extend your arms in front of you. Do not lock your elbows, but make sure all the muscles in your arms are engaged. Breathe in deeply through your nose, feeling your rib cage expand, and as you breathe out, feel your rib cage contract. Breathe several times in this position, then, keeping your fingers interlaced, lift your arms straight up above your head so that they are parallel with that imaginary string running from the top of your head. Simultaneously stretch your arms upward toward the ceiling and inward toward your ears. Hold there and inhale deeply, feeling your rib cage expand. Exhale, and feel your rib cage contract as your chest lowers. Repeat the breath several times.

Slowly bring your arms forward and hold them in front of you. Keeping the fingers interlaced, turn your palms toward you and reinterlace the fingers so that the pinky of the other hand is on the bottom. Repeat the steps above. (Incidentally, if you are right-handed, you probably unconsciously interlaced your hands so that the right pinky was on the bottom. This is just one of the unconscious ways we favor one side of the body over the other. You will probably notice throughout your yoga practice that you are stronger and more flexible on one side of the body than the other; yoga seeks to balance that imbalance.)

UJJAYI PRANAYAMA

The following breathing exercise enables you to slow down your rate of breathing. In a stressful situation the body's core temperature tends to drop as blood rushes to the extremities. *Ujjayi pranayama* counteracts this stress response, as the increased effort required to breathe in this fashion causes the body's core temperature to rise. In addition, when you breathe more slowly and with more control, you will be able to study your body and mind more acutely.

To prepare for this exercise you will need a bath towel that is rolled up lengthwise.

1. Place the rolled-up towel on the floor, then lie down upon it so that the towel lines up with your spine. One end of the towel should be at the base of your rib cage; the other end will probably extend beyond your head.

2. Blow air out from your mouth onto your open palm as if you were blowing bubbles through a ring. The air will seem cool and dry.

3. Now imagine that it is cold outside and that you want to see your breath. Constrict the muscles in the back of your throat and breathe out on your open palm. The air should now feel warmer and moister. (If you need another image, breathe out through your open mouth as if you were going to moisten your glasses before cleaning them.)

4. Retain that same feeling in the back of the throat that you feel when cleaning your glasses or seeing your breath in the winter, but now breathe out through your nostrils instead of through your mouth. Do you notice the accompanying echoing sound—it's a bit like the sound Darth Vader makes, right?

5. Once you have successfully felt and heard this breath on the exhale, see if you can discover it on the inhalation. This is a little harder. Make sure you are not "sniffing" your breath in—instead, imagine the breath entering horizontally more than vertically.

6. In the beginning you may be applying some effort to creating this special form of breathing. Make sure that you are not being forceful. Over time you will be able to refine this method of breathing: the sound will become more delicate, and the amount of effort involved will become minimal.

ASANA SERIES: REDUCING STRESS

The yoga practice on the following pages will help you deepen your overall awareness of your body, mind, and breath—one of the most important steps toward reducing stress. Sometimes flowing, sometimes static, this series of postures will help you explore the subtler layers of your being. Stay alert through the transitions into and out of each position—each *asana* builds upon the previous one.

You will be surprised how much of a change you will feel in your body as this series progresses. As you near the end of the practice, you will return to an *asana* practiced at the beginning of the series, and your body will likely stretch farther, without as much tension. Your muscles will be warmer and more pliable, and you will feel a connection between your body and your mind that is so often missing during daily life.

Be sure to remember your breathing as you move through these sometimes challenging positions. Maintaining full, complete breaths oxygenates your muscles and ensures that you achieve the full benefits of yoga practice. So focus on taking full, complete breaths in and out through your nostrils as you did in the breathing exercise on page 36. Concentrate on the soothing sound of your breath, and let it direct you inward to the flow of energy (or *prana*) coursing through your body. You cannot think your way into stress release; it is thoughts that are creating the stress you are trying to release. Go deeper than your thoughts, then, and let the breath initiate the movement into and out of the postures. Absorb the sensations.

Above all, in this series and in all the *asana* sequences in this book, be patient with yourself. The *asanas* are not exercises that need to be perfected. They are tools for self-exploration. The sequence provided here will let you experience your body in many different positions—

positions that you do not normally assume during the course of the day. You will be bending forward and backward, twisting right and left, and supporting your weight first with your leg strength and then with a combination of upper body and leg strength. Enjoy what you're doing! In each of the "situations" set up by a particular physical exercise, pay attention to the messages your body is sending you, and modify the posture if needed.

Practicing *asanas* asks for an approach that is different from the "no pain, no gain" approach of other exercise methods. The definition of an *asana*, according to Patanjali's *Yoga Sutras*, is *"shtira-sukham asanam,"* which means that unless the position is stable and practiced with comfort and ease, it is not an *asana*. On the outside you may "look" as if you are doing the pose "perfectly," but if you are struggling and straining on the inside, then refinement still needs to occur. The various alignment cues I have suggested are intended to help you move into, move out of, or stay in the pose safely; you are not locked into them, nor are they the secret to "perfecting" the posture.

You may find it challenging to achieve stability and ease in some of the postures. Going back to the *Sutras* again, Patanjali suggests that stability and ease may be found by relaxing our efforts and merging with our body's internal wisdom. This may seem antithetical to everything you have been taught or practiced in other environments—you may believe, for example, that the harder you work, the more comforts you will garner—but relaxed, mindful effort has been working for yogis for several thousand years now. An intrinsic comfort and stability exist inside you already; yoga practices are just tools to reveal them. Go ahead and trust your body's internal wisdom to direct you into the right alignment. Learn to let go. And when in doubt, return to your breathing and let go of your thinking.

ASANA SERIES

SUKHASANA

BREATH AWARENESS

CAT POSE TO CAT SEAL

CAT POSE TO DOWN DOG

MOVING THREE POINT

LUNGE FORWARD BEND

VIRABHADRASANA II TO SUPPORTED RIGHT ANGLE

UTKATASANA TO FORWARD BEND

CAT POSE TO CAT SEAL

SALABHASANA

CAT SEAL

MALTESE TWIST

RECLINED LEG EXTENSION

DANDASANA FORWARD BEND

VINYASA BRIDGE POSE

SAVASANA

SUKHASANA

SUKHASANA

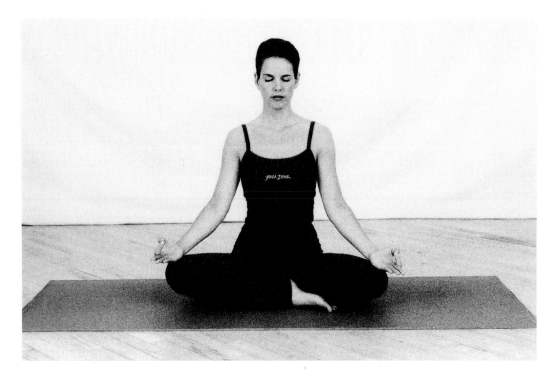

Sit cross-legged on the floor. Place your hands on your knees with the palms facing upward. Close your eyes, and feel where your energy is now. Are you feeling dull or tired, agitated or restless? Notice your breath. Is it short or shallow, deep or strained? Try not to judge your body or your breath—simply notice how you are feeling as you sit, supported by the knowledge that you will be moving forward from here.

BREATH AWARENESS

Initiate your breathing. When you inhale, become aware of an expansion in your body. Feel your rib cage expand and the top corners of your chest lift up. Feel your belly expand slightly as the diaphragm presses toward your lower abdomen.

When you exhale, feel your body contract. Gently pull in your lower abdomen, encouraging the expulsion of air from your core. Feel your rib cage and chest lower and relax.

Take six to eight full, complete breaths, noticing these subtle movements during inhalation and exhalation.

CAT POSE TO CAT SEAL

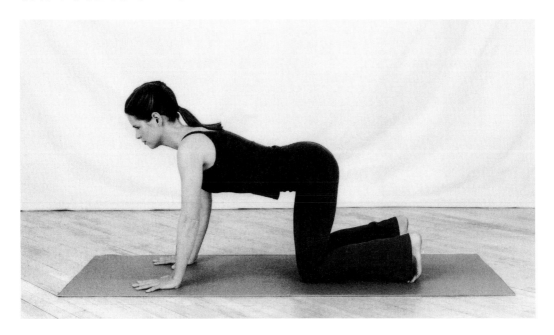

Slowly move to all fours, placing your knees under your hips and your hands beneath your shoulders. If your wrists are feeling tight, move your hands a bit forward or wider until they are comfortable. Spread your fingers, and position your hands so that the middle finger of each hand points forward. Inhale, and feel your rib cage expand, your torso elongate, and your spine draw in toward the core of your body. At the same time your shoulder blades move ever so slightly down your back, and your head lifts up. This is Cat Pose.

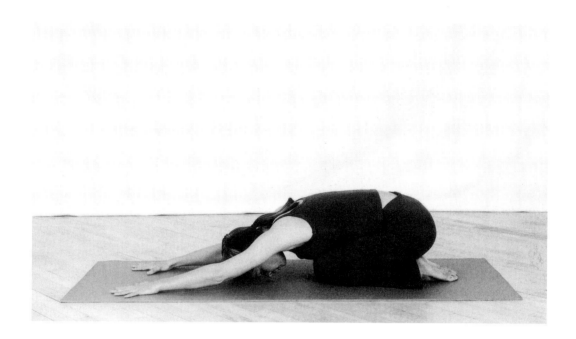

As you exhale, gently pull your lower abdomen in once again, and notice how your rib cage and chest contract as you move your body back toward your heels. This is Cat Seal. As you inhale again, let your breath expand your rib cage, and feel your chest and head move up and forward into Cat Pose. Then exhale, draw in your abdomen, and move back into Cat Seal. Repeat this movement several times.

CAT POSE TO DOWN DOG

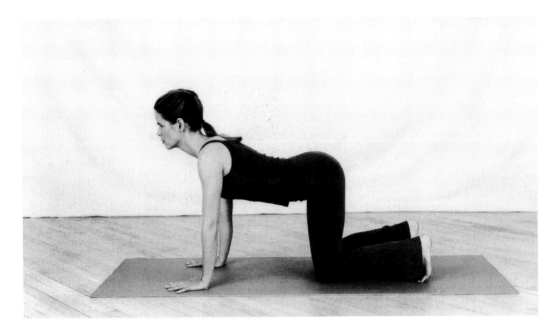

Once again feel yourself grounded on all fours, with your toes curled into the floor. As you inhale, expand your chest and ribs and move forward into Cat Pose.

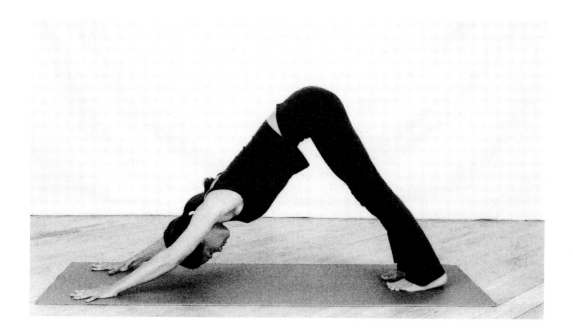

On the exhale, contract your thighs and lift your hips up as you draw in your abdomen. Be mindful of creating space between the tops of your shoulders and your head. Your heels move toward the floor and, together with your hands, create a stable base for the rest of your body. Picture yourself creating an upside-down V with your body. Maintain a slight bend in your knees as the backs of your legs stretch. This position is called Down Dog.

As you inhale, move forward into Cat Pose, then exhale once again into Down Dog. Repeat this movement several times.

MOVING THREE POINT

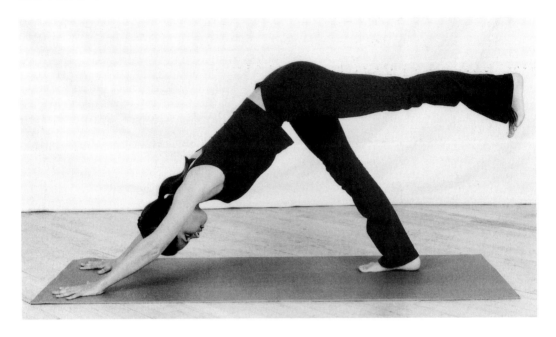

This next position is a moving variation of Down Dog. First, you need to establish a steady and solid Down Dog position. Keep your knees slightly bent, and check that your shoulders haven't dropped toward your ears. Check your arm position. Do not lock your elbow joints; instead, keep the elbows slightly bent, to make sure you are using your muscles, rather than your joints, to hold your weight. Then relax your head and neck. Make sure there is no tension in your jaw as you remain in Down Dog. Shake your head loosely back and forth as if you were saying yes and no, to ensure that no tension remains in your neck. Now you are ready to begin Moving Three Point.

On your next inhale, lift your left leg behind you. Keep your toes pointing toward the floor, and reach through the heel of your lifted leg. Try to feel your hips remaining even with each other and squared toward the front of your body. The tendency will be for your left hip to follow your leg into the air and rise much higher than the right hip. Resist this

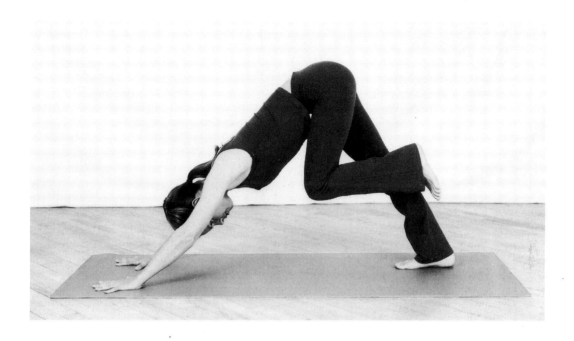

tendency, and keep both hips level. Once again feel the expansion of your chest and ribs. Your right leg should stay even with your sitting bones.

Next exhale, bend your left knee, and move your thigh toward your belly. Feel your ribs and chest contract and move toward the center of your body. Your head will follow.

Inhale, straighten the leg again, and reach through the heel. Your body follows the movement of your breath; your head, chest, and torso expand and move away from the center of your body. Repeat this movement three times, then switch to the right leg and do the same number of repetitions.

LUNGE FORWARD BEND

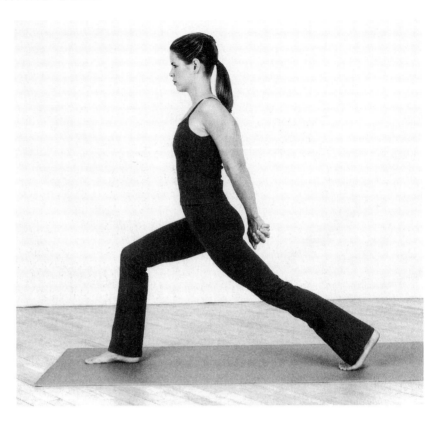

Stand with your feet hip distance apart. Step back on your left foot and bend your right knee, making sure it stays even with your ankle. If you have enough strength, keep your left leg straight; otherwise, lower the left knee to the floor. Do not allow your knee to move forward of your ankle. Adjust the width of your feet so that you feel stable. Keep both feet solidly on the ground and gently move your left hip forward to square with your right hip. Keep the back foot on the ground, bringing your weight to the outside of your back foot. Bring your arms behind your back, interlacing the fingers of your hands together.

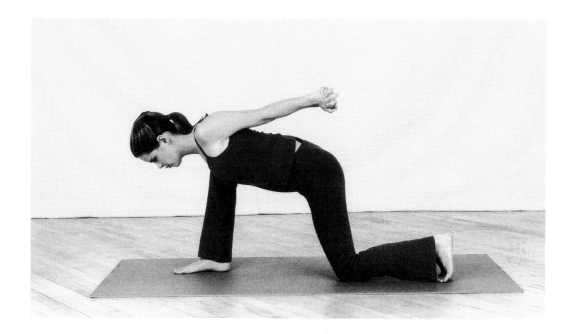

As you inhale, expand your chest and feel your spine lengthen. Try to keep your shoulders and neck relaxed. As you exhale, begin by drawing in your abdomen and bending forward from your hips. Keep length in your torso as you fold forward, releasing your head and neck when you reach your leg. On your inhale, use the strength of your legs and upper torso, as well as the expansion of your breath, to lift you back up into the position you started in. Do not initiate this motion from your lower back. Instead, keep tone in your abdomen and initiate the motion from your abdominal muscles. This will also help you keep your pelvis and hips in proper alignment.

As you exhale fold forward, then as you inhale rise back up. Repeat two more times, and then switch legs and do the other side for the same number of repetitions.

VIRABHADRASANA II TO SUPPORTED RIGHT ANGLE

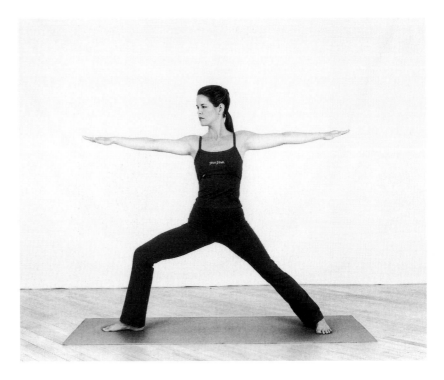

Stand with your feet a leg's length apart. Turn your left foot out to a 45-degree angle. Inhale, and feel your spine lengthen upward; when you exhale, bend your right knee to a 90-degree angle. On the next inhale raise your arms parallel to the floor, and when you exhale, feel the strength in your legs and abdomen. This is *Virabhadrasana* II. Stay for a couple of breaths to get comfortable with your alignment.

On an inhale, extend your right arm forward past your right knee. As you exhale, bend your right arm and place your forearm on your right thigh. This creates Supported Right Angle. Keep your front and back feet pressing firmly into the floor; do not transfer all your weight into that right arm.

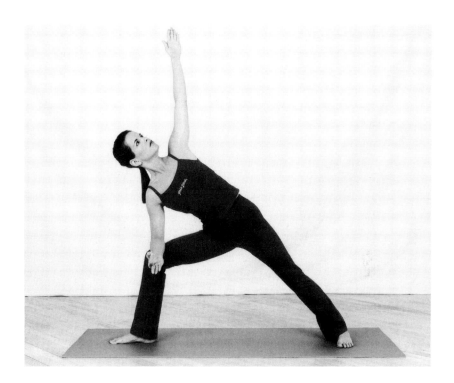

Once you feel established with the alignment of Supported Right Angle, move slowly back and forth between the two postures, letting your full, complete breaths move you from one to the other. Inhale to return to *Virabhadrasana* II, and when you exhale, slowly and gracefully move back into Supported Right Angle. Remember to feel the strength in your legs and abdomen, creating a firm base for the movements of your upper body.

This is a challenging sequence, but see if you can breathe comfortably while practicing four to six repetitions. After your last inhale returns you to *Virabhadrasana* II, exhale, straightening your right leg and lowering your arms alongside your torso. You are now ready, after a rest, to practice the sequence on the other side.

UTKATASANA TO FORWARD BEND

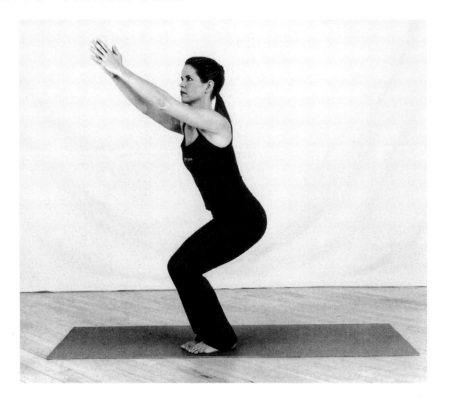

Stand with your feet a comfortable distance apart. As you inhale, bend your knees and raise your hands as high as you can without raising your shoulders. Pretend you are sitting in a chair. Use your leg muscles to hold your body as erect as possible. Feel an expansion in your chest and a lengthening through your spine to the crown of your head. This is *Utkatasana*.

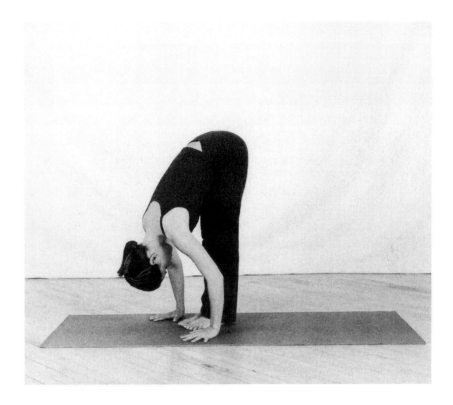

Next, initiate the exhale at your abdomen, pulling it in slightly. Let the contraction of your breath pull your torso up and forward, bending over toward your feet. Your arms will move with you, out and down to touch the floor or your shins.

As you inhale, begin at the top of the torso—be careful not to start with your lower back. Move forward and upward, back into *Utkatasana*. Exhale, and move forward and down into Forward Bend. Inhale, and move forward and up into *Utkatasana*. Repeat several times.

CAT POSE TO CAT SEAL

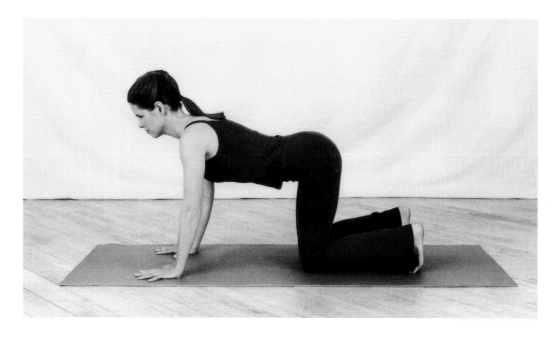

Practice this sequence (see pages 44–45) four to six times again, and observe how different it feels. Notice if your energy has changed and how. Do you feel less rigid, more flexible, or more alert? Is your body trying to send you any messages? Do you notice any remaining tension in your back or legs? Make note of these things, always noticing.

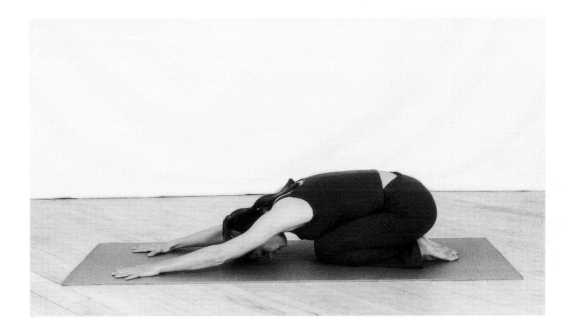

One goal of yoga is to bring you back into connection with your body, so that you notice from the beginning of your practice to the end how your muscles and joints are reacting to the postures. From one day to the next you will notice stress taking root differently in your body, or perhaps you will stop feeling physical tension altogether. It is all a matter of noticing. Yoga is a continual process of self-awareness—enjoy yourself.

SALABHASANA

Come now to lie flat on your belly. Your arms can lie alongside your torso with the palms of your hands facing down.

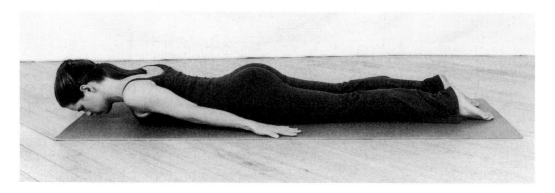

As you inhale, raise your torso and arms off the floor and look toward the ground. Resist the urge to carry tension in your face and jaw muscles—keep them relaxed. Focus on extending forward as much as on lifting up off the floor. Be careful as well not to shrug your shoulders up by your ears; rather, feel your shoulder blades drawing down your back.

Next, exhale, and lower your torso to the ground. Feel your rib cage pressing gently against the floor, helping to move the breath out of you. As you exhale, the upper back muscles that got shorter to lift you off the floor are now lengthening and lowering you back down to the ground. Rest for a moment.

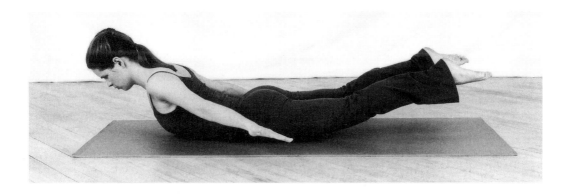

Now you are ready to add a lift of the legs. As you inhale, extend your legs backward and upward while lifting your arms and torso. It does not matter how high you lift your legs (or the rest of you for that matter!). Lower yourself on your exhalation. If you feel discomfort in your lower back, try imagining your tailbone pressing downward toward the floor as you lift up. You may also find additional support if your heels roll inward slightly. Practice this sequence of moving the legs, arms, and torso off the floor three times.

SALABHASANA (continued)

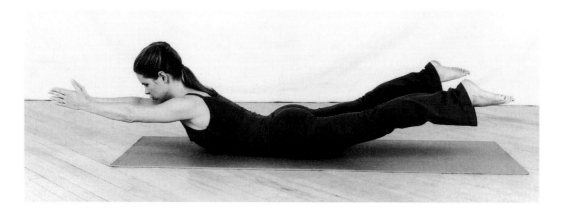

VARIATION: When raising your torso and legs, extend your arms in front of your body, palms facing each other, and separate your legs. This makes the pose considerably more challenging, but do not attempt it until you can hold the position comfortably while breathing fully and completely.

CAT SEAL

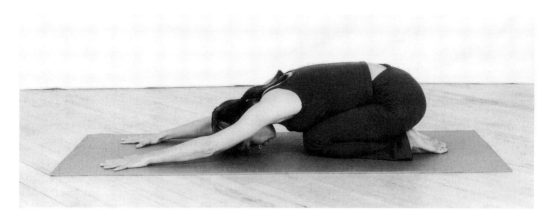

To rest after *Salabhasana,* press your seat backward onto your heels and come into Cat Seal (see page 45). This posture will stretch the muscles of your back and help to release any tension that may have accumulated. Do not expect to breathe deeply in this position, but do allow your breathing to expand the back of your body.

MALTESE TWIST

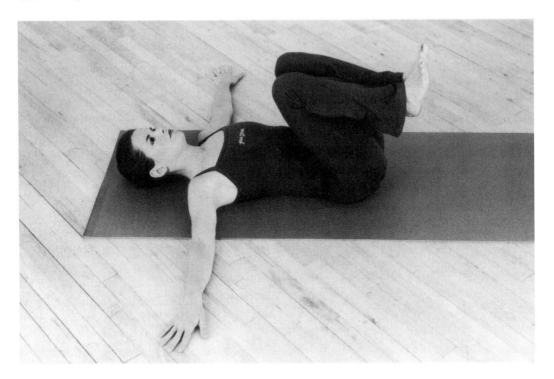

Come onto your back now. Lie flat with your knees bent and your arms outstretched but positioned a bit lower than your shoulders. Lift your hips a few inches off the floor, and while they are in the air, shift them over to the right side. Lower your hips. From this off-center position, bend your knees into your chest and let your legs drop over to the left side. (Note: You shifted your hips to the right side, but now you are dropping your knees over to the left side.)

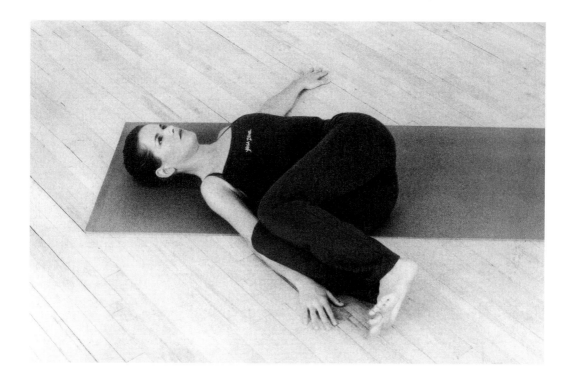

Your spine should now be lined up correctly—an imaginary line from the center of your pelvis to the center of your head should be straight. Your shoulders may not be flat against the floor—that's okay. Your lower back will be supported more if you can keep your knees stacked directly on top of each other. As you inhale, feel an extension along your spine, and on the exhale let your abdominal muscles contract and guide you into the twist. With every inhale feel length in your spine, and with every exhale explore to see if there is space inside to deepen your twist. After six to eight breaths, use an inhale to bring your legs off the floor and back up to your chest. Repeat the process to twist in the other direction.

RECLINED LEG EXTENSION

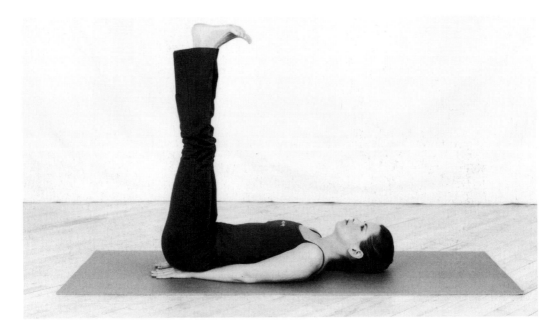

Continue to lie on your back with your knees pulled in toward your chest, but let your arms rest alongside your hips.

As you inhale, press your heels upward toward the ceiling. It is all right if you cannot completely straighten your legs; with time and practice you will improve.

As you exhale, bend your knees and draw your thighs back down toward your abdomen. Keep your lower back on the floor as you practice this breath-linked movement. As you breathe in and raise your heels, do not let your belly inflate—keep the breath in your chest. When you are drawing your knees in, feel as if your navel is being pressed by your exhale downward toward the floor. Repeat for six to eight breaths. When you have finished this sequence, roll onto your right side, then use your hands to press yourself up to a seated position.

DANDASANA FORWARD BEND

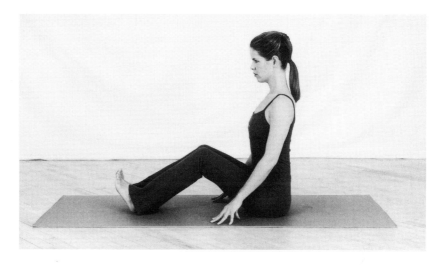

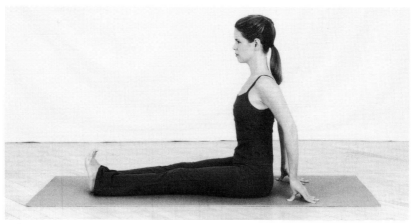

Stretch your legs out in front of you. Many people have tightness in their lower back or in the backs of their legs. In order to sit with your spine in an alignment that does not put excessive strain on your back and abdominal muscles, you will probably have to bend your knees slightly. Bending your knees will allow you to "perch" up on your sitting bones, the bony part of your seat. When your spine is properly aligned and your legs are outstretched, the *asana* is called *Dandasana.*

DANDASANA FORWARD BEND (continued)

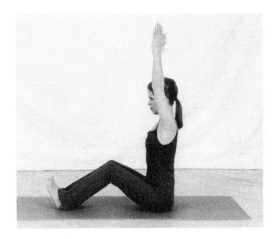 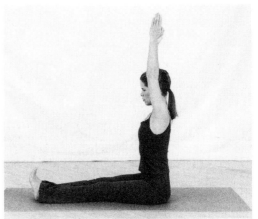

To move into *Dandasana* Forward Bend, raise your arms overhead on the inhale, and on the exhale rotate from your hips and extend your torso out over your legs. Your back should remain straight—make sure you are not bending from your waist or collapsing your chest over your legs. Your hands may not reach your feet, which is fine.

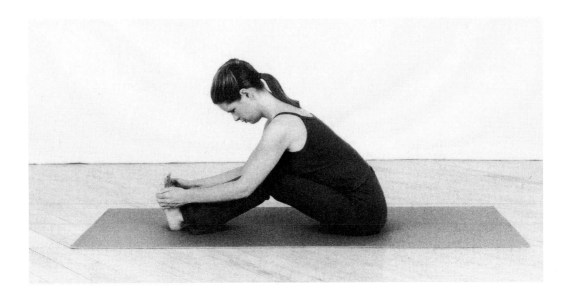

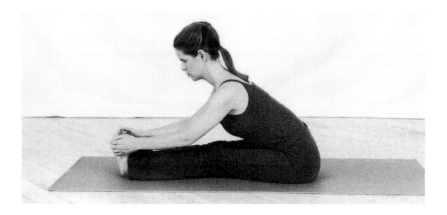

On an inhale reach your arms past your feet and draw your spine back up, starting from the back of your head, then the middle of your back. As you exhale, move back down into the forward bend. After three preparations stay in the forward bend, and notice how your breath affects the position. Do you ease more into the position as you exhale? Feel free to remain in *Dandasana* Forward Bend for six to eight breaths. To come out of the position, reach your arms past your feet, and on the inhale draw your spine back up and lower your arms alongside your torso.

VARIATION: As your back and abdominal muscles grow stronger, you may wish to try *Dandasana* Forward Bend with straighter legs

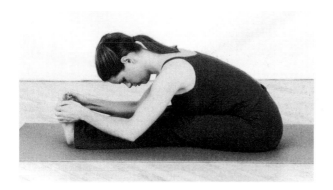

because you can achieve a deeper forward bend that way. You must make sure, however, that you are bending from your hips and that your back remains straight. It will do you no good to try this pose with straight legs if you are straining or rounding your back to touch your toes.

VINYASA BRIDGE POSE

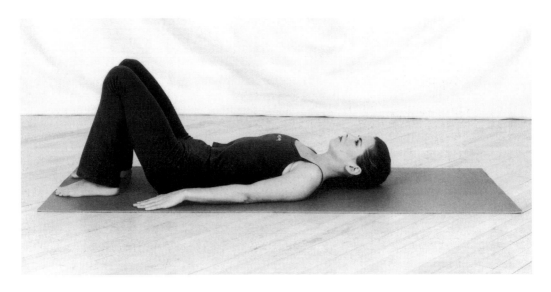

From a seated position, bend your knees and lower yourself down onto your back. Keep your knees bent. Adjust your feet so they are positioned more or less underneath your knees—how wide apart they are will be an individual matter. Experiment and make adjustments to keep your knees and lower back free of discomfort. Inhale, remaining on the floor and leaving your arms alongside.

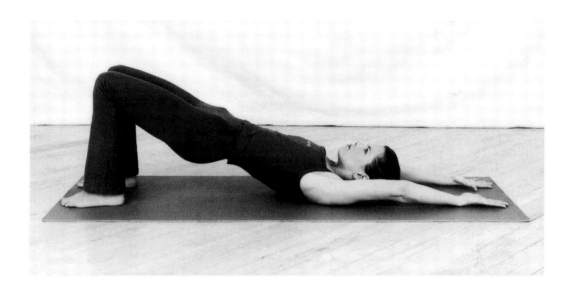

As you inhale, lift your hips off the floor by drawing your pelvis up toward your knees, away from your rib cage. You may raise your arms overhead and extend them to the floor behind you, as shown, or keep them alongside your body. As you exhale, keep your pelvis off the floor, then lower yourself down, first your upper back, then your midback, then place your lower back down, lowering your arms by your sides. Repeat this sequence four more times.

SAVASANA

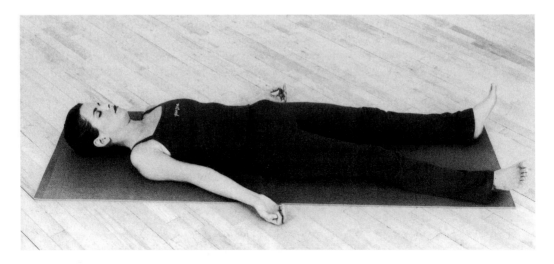

As you lie on the floor, extend your legs, letting your feet drop open in a way that feels comfortable to you. Draw your shoulder blades closer together and down your back so that your chest feels open and relaxed. Gently move your head from side to side until you find a comfortable resting position. Close your eyes, and observe your breathing without changing it. Try not to interfere with the inhalations or exhalations, and try not to disturb the pauses in between. Stay alert, but let go of the need to do anything. Remain here for as long as you like, but make sure you stay at least five minutes. There is no *asana* more satisfying after a yoga practice than *Savasana*.

SUKHASANA

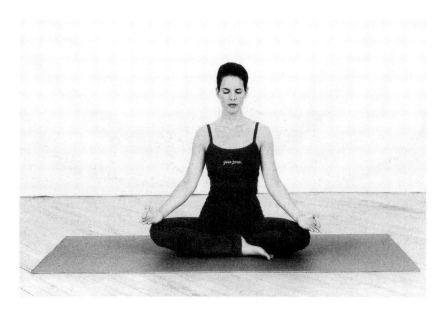

Come up to a cross-legged seat slowly so that the blood does not rush out of your head. Sit comfortably with your spine tall and your shoulders directly over your hips. Your knees should be slightly lower than the tops of your hips; if they are not, you may need some padding underneath your sitting bones to elevate your torso. Sit with your heels lined up, one in front of the other; if your heels do not line up, line up your ankles or shins instead. If sitting in a chair is better on your back or knees, please make that modification. Once you have found a position that you can maintain for five minutes, rest the backs of your hands on your knees and close your eyes.

VARIATIONS ON THIS *ASANA* SERIES

Before you begin your physical practice, quiet your mind with the practice of *pranayama*. Try *ujjayi pranayama* (see page 36), Alternate Nostril Breathing (see page 151), or the *Kriya* Yoga Breath (see page 153).

Pick a *kosha* (see page 93), and focus your *asana* practice upon it.

Follow this *asana* practice with a meditation on the chakras (see page 98), to create balance between them. Meditate for a few minutes on the *mantra* (sound) and *yantra* (shape) that correspond to each of the seven chakras. Or if you prefer, pick one chakra, and focus your attention solely on its *mantra* and *yantra.*

MEDITATION

The meditation technique *Prana Ahuti Kriya* is simple, yet requires supreme concentration and discipline. You must sit as still as a statue, resisting any temptation to move, fidget, scratch, or realign yourself in any way. Remain perfectly still. Do, however, allow your body to relax; this is not a rigid posture. Allow the subtle movements of your breathing to be the only physical movements you make. Let the breath adjust to this stillness. At first it may be uneven, or you may sigh or inhale deeply. As tension releases from your body, however, you will be inclined toward deeper and deeper stillness. When the breath becomes quiet and longer pauses have naturally developed in between inhales and exhales, feel as if a golden stream of light were flooding downward upon you, through the top crown of your head, filling your spine, and creating an oasis of warm golden light at the base of your spine. Let this light pour into you and fill each and every cell of your body until you are brimming over with light and warmth. Remain in this state for as long as it is comfortable.

To come out, drop your chin down into your chest and allow your breath rate to increase gradually. Slowly let your eyes crack open, and become aware of your surroundings. Stretch your legs out, and take some time to integrate into the room before moving on to your next activity.

3

MOVING YOGA OFF THE MAT

From contentment, unsurpassed happiness is gained.

PATANJALI, *YOGA SUTRAS*, CHAPTER 2, VERSE 42

THE BEGINNING YOGA PRACTITIONER SOON LEARNS THAT YOGA'S BENEFITS ARE NOT DISCOVERED ONLY BETWEEN THE FOUR WALLS OF THE STUDIO OR ON THE STICKY MAT. MUCH MORE THAN JUST A FABULOUS WORKOUT, YOGA IS best known for lengthening, strengthening, and defining the muscles, improving posture, providing gentle cardiac exercise, and increasing flexibility while decreasing the daily stress that often burrows into the body and takes residence there. But while yoga practitioners enjoy continual improvement in their bodies, physical conditioning is only the first benefit of practicing yoga with discipline and regularity.

With regular yoga practice, you will most likely begin to view life's inevitable challenges with serenity, and you will have a healthier context for dealing with emotional stress. Your daily life will be infused with the peaceful energy and harmony that are the mark of a productive, balanced yoga session. Some of your new-found serenity will be conscious: perhaps when you are in an argument, you will notice yourself taking shallow breaths, and you deliberately make a concerted effort to lengthen and deepen your breathing, a process that will evaporate stress. Other mental benefits will be unconscious. A fundamental sense of peace comes from achieving control over your body and breath and from knowing that you have the ability to focus and control your thoughts and reduce your physical stress. You may not even notice the new peacefulness that descends upon your life until you realize that this feeling of well-being never seems to dissipate, as it did before when you were confronted with stress or difficult decisions.

Yoga is not a religion, although at times it may feel as all-encompassing as religion. Yoga is and always has been an entirely secular science of health, wellness, and mental and physical discipline. Its practice does not conflict with any religion; nor does one have to be religious to practice yoga.

How can yoga be all-encompassing? The physical and mental awareness you enjoy after a yoga class may remain with you for a few hours or even for a few days. But when you carry that awareness into your daily activities, you are practicing yoga—even if you are not working on an *asana* on your sticky mat. You will find that you can practice yoga in many many different situations just by waking up the senses in your dealings with others and with the world that surrounds you.

YOGA AT THE GROCERY STORE

Believe it or not, with a slight change in perspective, you can even turn a visit to the grocery store into a yoga practice. To define an activity as yoga, you need only address it with the same awareness and consciousness as you address *asanas, pranayama,* and meditation during the practice hour. You can do this just as easily in the grocery store as in the studio!

First, notice how you use your body as you walk down the aisles and fill your cart. Are you standing tall, or are you hunched over the basket? Are you leaning to one side? Are you tense in any part of your body? When you bend forward to get something off a bottom shelf, is there a consciousness to your movement, or are you straining your back muscles? Do your movements emphasize one side of your body over the other? Do you reach out with your right arm more often than your left?

All these actions leave their mark on your body. If you hunch over a grocery cart as you shop, your back muscles will work harder than if you were standing straight. Next time you practice a back bend on your mat, you will feel the tension and wonder where it came from. Over time slouching can lead to irrevocably bad posture. So practicing standing straight behind a grocery cart can have effects as positive as a rigorous hour of yoga.

Continue your grocery store yoga practice by observing your breathing. Breathing is an unconscious process—luckily, so you can continue to do it even when confronted with outside distractions! Before you make a selection, try taking a long breath through your nose, deep into your lungs. Feel the top corners of your chest lifting and your rib cage expanding. Do you add the item to your cart after taking a moment to breathe? Later, as you stand in the express checkout line behind someone with more than ten items, notice your breathing. Is it tight and shallow? Is it worth getting upset over this? Examine your thoughts, and try lengthening your breath. It is better to enjoy the extra few moments in the checkout line than to fret over them.

Finally, notice the movements of your mind as you proceed through the store. Grocery stores are designed to stimulate the senses and inspire you to buy things, not necessarily to help you focus on what you need. Notice all the distractions that draw your attention away from conscious shopping and from your grocery list. Observe the smells, the sounds, the visual displays, and the tasting opportunities; touch the produce, squeeze the toilet paper, and flip through magazines at the checkout. Do your senses inspire you to act in habitual, unconscious ways, or do you discover new things? When you leave the store, do you feel that your shopping experience has been more complete? Do you feel a sense of contentment, or do you have any regrets?

Viewing a trip to the grocery store in this way may seem a bit comical, but the larger purpose is to show you the normal lack of awareness in routine activities such as shopping. Nonetheless, an awareness of movement, breath, thoughts, and your relationship to the world can bring you true happiness and serenity. Practice conscious breath, movement, and thought in all your waking activities, and you are practicing yoga.

Yoga in Your Relationships with Others

THERE'S NO DENYING IT: relationships with other people can cause stress. Sometimes at the height of an argument or misunderstanding, people get so agitated that it can be difficult to understand exactly what issues are at hand and how to regain balance and harmony. When the agitation of the moment is gone, however, your perception of the discord can become much clearer. This is the reason people count to ten before responding in a heated situation!

In many ways, the mindset of yoga is similar to "counting to ten" because it provides the necessary perspective to understand the body's reactions to outside influences. It provides the means to analyze and correct unnecessary negative reactions by placing them in a larger context. This kind of calm, reasoned consideration makes it easier to understand the stress that really matters and the stress that we can easily shed.

More concretely, if you feel that being around a particular person (let's call him Tom) always makes you angry, and you want to understand why your relationship with Tom creates anger, you will need to examine the three most basic components of that relationship: yourself, Tom, and the way you and Tom are linked. The main problem with a stress-causing relationship is that it emotionally distracts you from the effortless focus and understanding that are the goal and heart of yoga. Surprisingly, asking some very basic questions can often lead to a more sophisticated understanding of the relationship, releasing the strong emotions that lie within: How do you perceive Tom? How are you listening to Tom? How does Tom talk to you? How do you respond—outwardly *and* inwardly—when you begin to feel anger? Does the anger come from you originally, or does it originate from Tom? Is the anger simply a result of our interaction, or are there larger issues at hand?

Asking these questions about your relationship with Tom is a yoga practice in and of itself. Since anger is a distraction that gets in the way of focused attention, use that energy to fuel further exploration of who you are and how you are relating with the world around and inside you. No technique will enable you to change Tom, to make him into someone who does not anger you, but yoga's various tools (*asanas, pranayama,* meditation) can put you in better touch with yourself (as the subject) and make you aware of how you are linking with the objects around and inside you. To the extent that self-awareness is limited, a physical yoga practice enables you to expand your sense of identity because it requires you to give attention to your body, mind, and breath. Developing a broader perspective on the yoga mat will translate into a broader perspective off the mat: it is the same introspective process, whether you apply it to an *asana* or to your relationship with Tom.

The more clarity (the Sanskrit word is *viveka*) you can bring to your relationships, the less stressful they will be. The more you fine-tune your awareness of your emotional connection to others, the more you will be able to approach every relationship in your life as if it were a mirror reflecting back valuable information about where you stand spatially, physically, emotionally, spiritually, and philosophically from moment to moment. You'll be able to view your relationships from all angles to make sure you aren't missing anything important. You will be a better, more observant friend because you will listen and understand as never before.

RELATIONSHIP MEDITATION

According to Patanjali's *Yoga Sutras,* there are four kinds of behavior that we are likely to encounter throughout the course of our day: behavior characterized by comfort or ease, behavior characterized by pain or sorrow, behavior that is virtuous, or behavior that is nonvirtu-ous. How we relate to those behaviors—which may be found in oth-ers or in ourselves—will influence whether they disrupt the balance and harmony within us.

Yoga provides the following behavior "couplings" to create harmony:

TOWARD PEOPLE OR SITUATIONS THAT ARE . . .	PRACTICE . . .
COMFORTABLE (SUKHA)	FRIENDLINESS (MAITRI)
PAINFUL (DUKHA)	COMPASSION (KARUNA)
VIRTUOUS (PUNYA)	JOYFULNESS (MUDITA)
NOT VIRTUOUS (APUNYA)	NOT DIRECTING YOUR ENERGY TOWARD THEM (UPEKSHANAM)

It is probably easy to list people and situations in your life that can be characterized by the words in the left column. If you notice that you have a hard time interacting with people who illustrate those four qualities, you can counteract the discomfort by meditating on the Sanskrit word for the associated practice. For instance, if you find it difficult to be happy when others are happy, then throughout the day or at the end of a meditation practice silently recite the Sanskrit word *maitri* (pronounced *my-tree*) to yourself. If other people's (or your own!) difficulties irritate you, use *karuna* (pronounced *car-roon-a*). Or if per-haps you are jealous of other people's virtues or self-conscious of your own, repeating *mudita* (pronounced *mood-ie-tah*) will trigger a change in you. And lastly, if you sense yourself being distracted at times by oth-ers' or your own lack of virtue, link your attention to *upekshanam* (pro-nounced *oo-peck-sha-num*).

YOGA OF THE SENSES

Our five senses—taste, touch, sight, smell, and hearing—allow us to experience the physical, material world in which we live. As you have learned in your yoga practice, the sensory world is important, but there are other levels of perception as well, which are there for us if we can move past the limitations of our senses. Taking time to experience each sense and understand its effect upon you can be a valuable lesson in thoughtful concentration. This in turn will have a remarkable effect upon your yoga practice.

Have you ever given much thought to how your senses shape you? Often, our five senses are overloaded by strong stimuli competing for our attention. Think about it. Does the visual appeal of television advertising create desires for objects you don't really want? Does the taste of certain foods create unhealthy appetites and cause you to overeat needlessly? Or, on a positive note, can a calming piece of music quiet your mind, relax your body, and improve your practice of the *asanas*? These are all examples of the senses affecting your life in ways that you may not have given careful attention—until now.

Yoga is a tradition of experiences, and understanding how your senses shape your experience of the material world can help you open the door to higher perception. The more you learn to be conscious and aware in your sensory life, the more passionate your yoga practice will be. Below are some exercises to help you thoughtfully consider your five senses. These exercises will help heighten your awareness, and as you bring your new perspective on sight, touch, smell, sound, and hearing to your daily life, you may find that you are less bonded to the physical world and to the unhealthy and often unfulfilled desires it can sometimes create.

Work with one sense at a time, and spend at least ten minutes on each. Do not overload yourself with all five in one sitting. You are probably not used to this kind of focused concentration. This is training. Give yourself time to develop the skills.

TASTE

How many times have you sat down at the dinner table and mindlessly eaten a meal, paying more attention to the dinner conversation or to the thoughts swirling through your head than to the food you are eating? As with the grocery store practice, you can create a yoga practice by tuning your mind to your sensation of taste.

Taste is perhaps the most local of the senses. Tastes, whether salty, bitter, pungent, sour, or sweet, are perceived on the tongue and influenced by the sense of smell. Until an object enters your mouth, you have no taste-related information about it. As soon as the information comes in, it is immediately influenced by memory and intellect. The associations we develop around taste are especially volatile. With frequent exposure to one taste over another, we develop preferences. These preferences exist in the mind but are not necessarily correlated elsewhere. Does your body prefer an excess of sweet and salty foods? Does it perform better on a diet consisting solely of pungent foods? Does your body crave a particular taste, or does your mind crave it? Have you lost the ability to taste—how aware are you of fully tasting something? Have you ever given serious thought to how your senses shape and mold you?

The Tantric master Bharati used to prescribe exercises to heighten awareness of the senses. He insisted that the more alive the senses were, the more passionate one would be in the practice of yoga. The exercise that follows is an adaptation of Bharati's tasting exercise. You can adapt it as you see fit. The intention is to help you become more aware of your sense of taste.

The exercise requires a bit of preparation. In advance, gather representatives of the five tastes (salty, sweet, sour, pungent, and bitter). Spices often provide the most "pure" experiences. Try using salt, sugar, lemon, ground mustard, and baker's chocolate, respectively.

PRACTICING TASTE

1. Sit comfortably and close your eyes.
2. Without placing anything in your mouth, become aware of the tastes that are already there. They may change throughout the course of the exercise. Keep your jaw relaxed, your teeth apart, the roof of your mouth soft, and the back of your throat open.
3. After a few minutes, place one of the tastes in your mouth. Try not to identify it in advance. (It may help to have the spices on spoons—choose randomly.)
4. Try to stay with the experience. Do not be in a rush to get on to the next taste. How does the taste change over time?
5. Repeat with the four other tastes.
6. Afterward, note what thoughts, sensations, and feelings came up. What, if anything, kept you from fully tasting any of the different tastes?

SIGHT

Sight is perhaps the most obvious of the senses, because it provides us with the greatest amount of information. From the moment you open your eyes each morning, your brain is barraged by an assortment of colors and shapes on which you form opinions. We all have individual aesthetic preferences; we build ourselves beautiful homes to live in and surround ourselves with objects we find beautiful. But does visual beauty bring true happiness? Not really. How often do you let aesthetics shape your perception of worth?

Sight is also often metaphorically used to indicate understanding. When we finally grasp a difficult concept, we exclaim, "Oh, I see!" But seeing and understanding are not as linked as the metaphor suggests. Yoga teaches us that there are levels of understanding beyond the physical senses that we must strive to achieve. In fact, one of the first steps of any meditation practice is to close one's eyes and filter out the visual distractions that inhibit higher-level consciousness.

By spending a few minutes meditating on your sense of vision you may find you have a better understanding of how it affects your perception of the world around you. Here is an exercise to help you explore the sense of sight.

PRACTICING SIGHT

1. Sit comfortably (cross-legged or in a straight-backed chair) in a quiet location that is familiar to you—a garden or a favorite room, perhaps. Let the backs of your hands rest comfortably on the tops of your thighs or knees.

2. Keep your eyes open, and softly gaze toward a central point. Let the muscles around your eyes soften, and allow your vision to

become panoramic. It's okay to blink if you need to, but try not to move at all other than that. Let the images come to you and imprint themselves on your consciousness without your describing to yourself what is happening.

3. After ten minutes note what thoughts, sensations, or feelings came to you during this meditation. Note the distractions that came in the way of your seeing.

SMELL

Smell is one of the subtler of the five senses. There are times when you may not even be fully conscious of the mild smells you are perceiving. We humans don't use our sense of smell to interpret the world to the extent that other species do, and so, as with the sense of sound, there are subtle distinctions of smell that we often fail to notice.

Spend a few minutes thinking about your sense of smell and how it affects your perception of the world around you. Are there any smells you have not fully noticed? How do they affect you? Here is an exercise to help you explore the sense of smell.

PRACTICING SMELL

1. Choose a location that has some distinctive smells (a garden, your kitchen). Sit comfortably, and close your eyes.
2. Let the smells be drawn into your nose.
3. Are there layers of smell? Are there multiple smells?
4. After ten minutes note what thoughts, sensations, and feelings came to you during this meditation. Note the distractions that came in the way of your smelling.

HEARING

We all know that loud, grating, or sudden sounds may inhibit our ability to focus and build awareness, but gentler sounds may actually aid concentration. A CD of quiet natural sounds or music can be a valuable addition to any yoga practice; Yoga Zone has a good collection, including *Yoga Zone Ocean of Peace, Yoga Zone Garden of Peace, Yoga Zone Music for Meditation,* and *Yoga Zone Music for Practice.*

And remember, some sounds are easier to hear than others. It's hard to miss the blaring horns of rush hour traffic or the roar of a train, but there may be other sounds that are less perceptible. Spend a few minutes thinking about your sense of hearing and how it affects your perception of the world around you. Are there any sounds you do not listen closely enough to hear? Here is an exercise that will help you explore the sense of hearing. It is best practiced in a fairly quiet room.

PRACTICING HEARING

1. Sit comfortably, and close your eyes.
2. Bring your awareness to all the sounds that are outside of you. After a while shift your attention to all the sounds that are inside you.
3. After ten minutes note the thoughts, sensations, and feelings that came up during this meditation. Note the distractions that came in the way of your hearing.

TOUCH

If you've practiced meditation, you know how the sense of touch affects your connection to the physical world, even when you have been successful in quieting the other senses. Here is an experience that may sound all too familiar: You've sat down in a room free of distracting noises, closed your eyes, and begun to focus your attention on your breathing and to quiet your mind for meditation. But the floor you are sitting on is too hard! It's difficult to draw your attention away from that discomfort, isn't it? And then, what about that itch on your foot? These tactile distractions are constant reminders of the physical world, and it can be a challenge to filter them out.

Spend a few minutes thinking about your sense of touch and how it affects your perception of the world around you, not only during meditation but during the course of your entire day. Here is an exercise to help you explore the sense of touch.

PRACTICING TOUCH

1. Close your eyes.
2. Bring your awareness to everything that is touching you. Observe the gross objects that you are in contact with (the floor, the ground, the chair). Gradually bring your awareness to the subtler things, such as your clothes, or a breeze against your skin. Absorb these touches through every pore of your skin without moving. If itches come, let them stay unscratched. If you are outside and bugs land on you, try to let them touch you without reacting.
3. After ten minutes note what thoughts, sensations, and feelings came to you during this meditation. Note the distractions that came in the way of your touch.

Heightening your senses will increase your capacity for desire. Learn to distinguish between the desires of the material world and the desires of yoga. Retailers, for example, are sophisticated in the art of stimulating the senses to heighten customers' desire for a quick fix. Vibrant colors, delicious smells, pleasant sounds, sensual strokes, and sweet tastes are all employed to fuel the culture of commercial desire. The idea that the fulfillment of these desires will bring you true happiness is just an illusion *(maya)*. Try to increase your ability to move past temporary desires—they are just distractions on your path to ultimate enlightenment.

For Further Exploration

IF YOU WISH TO LEARN more about yoga and meditation, you may be interested in the following works.

BOOKS

The Anatomy Coloring Book, Wynn Kapit and Lawrence M. Elson
(Benjamin/Cummings, 2001)

Anatomy of Movement, Blandine Calais-Germain
(Eastland Press, 1993)

Autobiography of a Yogi, Paramahansa Yogananda
(Self Realization Fellowship Pub., 1979)

Ayurveda: The Ancient Indian Healing Art, Scott Gerson, M.D.
(Element Books, 1993)

The Bhagavad Gita, translated by Winthrop Sargeant
(State University of New York Press, 1994)

Light on Yoga, B.K.S. Iyengar
    (Schocken Books, 1995)

The Shambala Encyclopedia of Yoga, Georg Feuerstein, Ph.D.
    (Shambala, 1997)

Wheels of Life: A User's Guide to the Chakra System, Anodea Judith, Ph.D.
    (Llewellyn Publications, 1987)

The Yoga Sutras of Patanjali, translated by Sri Swami Satchidananda
    (Integral Yoga Distribution, 1990)

Yoga Zone Introduction to Yoga, Alan Finger with Al Bingham
    (Three Rivers Press, 2000)

CDs

Life Enhancing Meditations by Alan Finger
    (Relaxation Company, 2003)

Yoga Zone Garden of Peace
    (BMG Entertainment, 1998)

Yoga Zone Music for Meditation
    (BMG Entertainment, 1998)

Yoga Zone Music for Practice
    (BMG Entertainment, 1998)

Yoga Zone Ocean of Peace
    (BMG Entertainment, 1998)

4

DISCOVERING THE SELF

All confusion about the nature of the Self vanishes
for one who has seen its glory.

PATANJALI, *YOGA SUTRAS*, CHAPTER 4, VERSE 25

ONE OF THE MOST ENLIGHTENING PARTS OF YOGA PRACTICE IS THE NEW PERSPECTIVE IT GIVES YOU. AS YOU PROBE DEEPER INTO THE THEORY BEHIND YOUR PHYSICAL PRACTICE, YOU WILL FIND YOURSELF CONSIDERING YOUR OWN identity and your relationship to the world around you in entirely different ways.

The concept of the "self" in yoga departs from the ideas about identity that you probably have learned for your whole life. Yoga theory holds that every conscious person has two parts of the self: *jiva-atman* and *param-atman*. Your *jiva-atman* can be considered to be your individual personality, which is shaped by your feelings and your relationship to the sensory world. It is tied to the material world and forms its tastes and preferences—its identity—based on the duality of that world. Hot and cold, sweet and sour, high and low—these opposites allow us to find our way through the world, using taste, touch, sight, smell, and hearing. But those senses have little to do with the higher questions every human being grapples with: Who am I? Why am I here? What is my place in the world? Yet many people get caught up in the material world and come to base their identities upon it (a woman who is known for her great fashion sense, for example, or a man who will only eat the best gourmet food). But those sorts of identities, we all know, deep down, are very superficial. By defining ourselves in those sensory ways, we close ourselves off to the larger parts of our consciousness.

You may find answers to those overarching life questions—Who am I? Why am I here? What is my place in the world?—or at least a new way of considering them, in the idea of *param-atman*, the other part of the self. Your *param-atman*, which is unfettered from the sensory world, deals in inspiration, intuition, and insight. It is the part of your consciousness that can identify with a greater universal consciousness. It is the part of you that recognizes something wise and wonderful in the universe and strives to understand it.

So now that you understand that you have a *param-atman*, how do you access that wonderful new part of your consciousness? It will require some effort.

A barrier exists between your sensory self (*jiva-atman*) and your higher consciousness (*param-atman*). It is made up of the beliefs you have been forming ever since you were born, beliefs that are grounded in the sensory world. These beliefs, in Sanskrit, are called *avidya*.

The problem with *avidya* is that it blocks our ability to be aware of our ability to be aware. Let's untangle that thought! Metaphorically speaking, being blocked by *avidya* is like walking outside into a cloudy day. The skies are gray, light cannot pierce through the clouds, and those things affect your ability to perceive the world around you. You may not face the world as clearly or as cheerfully as you would on a day when the weather was nicer. You may make the wrong decision because your perception is "clouded."

Becoming aware of your *param-atman* is like the sun coming out, or turning on a light. You become exposed to intuition, inspiration, and insight. But how can the physical practice of yoga give you such mental clarity? How can it help you get in touch with your *param-atman?*

The answer is both simple and very complex. The fact is, the very discipline your yoga practice requires of you helps you become aware of *param-atman* and your essential connection to the universe. At the end of each *asana* practice, you relax in corpse position. During that time your cells act as tiny sponges, absorbing the intuition, insight, and inspiration of the universe. You will feel it then, and you will bring it into your daily life. The clouds will part, you will recognize the limits of *avidya,* and even more important, you will realize your intimate connection with the universe.

An Expanded Definition of the Self: The *Koshas*

FOR LACK OF A BETTER IDEA, many people equate the "self" with its physical manifestation—the touchable, fleshy, external body. But yoga teaches us and allows us to experience that there are five sheaths, or *koshas,* that make up the self. Unlike the tiers on a wedding cake or the rings of an onion, the *koshas* are not easy to separate and label; they overlap and intermingle. Metaphorically, this mingling is similar to the ingredients in a fruit smoothie. When you put a smoothie together, you know that it has different components— orange juice, pineapple juice, a banana, yogurt, honey, and so on. But once those ingredients are blended together, it is much more difficult to look at the smoothie and identify its parts. At the same time, when you taste it, you can easily recognize the different intermingled flavors.

So it is with the *koshas.* Combined, they are difficult to recognize, but with practice we can learn to "taste" their presence.

Defining the Five *Koshas* and Focusing the *Asana* Practice upon Them

DO NOT BE ALARMED if the concept of the *koshas* seems strange to you at first. As in the smoothie metaphor, we experience these different elements on a daily basis in a mixed-together way. To begin to sense the separate sheaths of the self, you may wish to focus your *asana* practice on one *kosha* at a time. To vary your practice from day to day, you may focus any of the *asana* series in this book on one *kosha.* Some suggestions on how to do that follow.

ANNOMAYA KOSHA

The densest, most solid aspect of the being is *annomaya kosha,* roughly translated as "food-body." *Annomaya kosha* is made up of the food we eat. It is the physical body, the flesh, muscle, blood, and bones.

Here is a practice focused on *annomaya kosha:*

I. As you assume the different postures, become absorbed in the structure that is holding you together.

2. Be particularly conscious of your body's alignment and how it changes from moment to moment.

3. Recognize that your body is in continual motion, even when still.

4. Explore each pose while taking in the whole of your body; do not limit your attention to the particular part of the body, such as the thighs or the arms, that seems to be doing the most "work."

PRANAMAYA KOSHA

Pranamaya kosha is the energy sheath. This part of the self comprises all energy transactions in the body, such as blood flow, oxygen absorption, and neurochemical impulses. *Prana,* translated as "life force," exists not only in the body but all around it as well. When two clouds bump into each other during a storm, *prana* is expressed as lightning. Since *pranamaya kosha* is not confined to the physical body, you may sense it around you as well, especially after meditation or *asana* practice. It feels like a glow, a warmth; some people refer to it as an aura. When your practice begins to open up energy flow within the body, people may begin to detect a glow around you, a new-found brilliance to your appearance. This is *pranamaya kosha* revealing itself.

Here is a practice focused on *pranamaya kosha:*

1. Recognize that you are an energetic being. *Prana,* life force, enters on your breath, responsible for every function that happens within you.

2. Practice the *asanas* with the knowledge that every cell of your body is breathing. Feel the expansion with every inhalation and the contraction with every exhalation.

3. Try relaxing your effort, and let your body breathe on its own as you move through the postures. Let your body tell you how much oxygen, and how much *prana,* it needs for each position.

MANOMAYA KOSHA

Manomaya kosha is the mental and emotional experiences that are contained within your self. Your experiences shape you. The way you speak, your mannerisms, the way you sneeze, laugh, and cry, even the way you walk into a room—all those things have been shaped by experience, by particular thoughts that happened so long ago you can no longer remember them. Since many thoughts, habits, and actions are unconscious, *manomaya kosha* can be very difficult to identify. But developing an awareness of this layer is crucial to self-exploration and transformation.

Here is a practice focused on *manomaya kosha:*

1. As you practice, let the mind serve you. Don't be at the beck and call of your thoughts.

2. Now put your mind in charge of a task, one task, and see to what extent it is able to hold that task in its attention throughout the practice. For example, decide that you are going to create equal inhalations and exhalations. Inhale for three seconds, then exhale for three seconds. Try to keep your mind aware of maintaining equal inhales and exhales in the face of any distractions that may come up.

3. If you notice your mind wandering, gently bring it back without feeling that you have done anything wrong. Just pick up the exercise where you left off.

VIJNANAMAYA KOSHA

Vijnanamaya kosha is the sheath of innate intelligence. Some of the things that you know, you had to be taught—the alphabet, how to count, how to multiply, how to pray. But you came into this world already knowing how to breathe, how to digest food, and how to eliminate toxins from the body. This intelligence resides in *vijnanamaya kosha.* The same innate intelligence also encompasses your natural inclinations or talents—to be a dancer, or a doctor, or a teacher. Your ability to access *vijnanamaya kosha* and understand your natural tendencies depends wholly on the permeability of *annomaya, pranamaya,* and *manomaya koshas.* If tension or distress is present in the other sheaths, you may not be as easily able to awaken your innate intelligence.

Here is a practice focused on *vijnanamaya kosha:*

1. Your body can find the "right" alignment for the poses using its innate intuition. Your breathing will happen even without your involvement. Throughout your practice, experiment with applying effort or surrendering to an "inner knowledge" of the postures.
2. Abandon the "proper" way of doing the poses, and instead listen to your body's needs. Discover the poses as if for the first time.
3. How does approaching the practice this way change your perception of the series?

ANANDAMAYA KOSHA

Anandamaya kosha is the core of our being, the bliss sheath, encompassing the capacity we all have to experience boundless joy. The awareness of bliss is *samadhi,* which we discussed in Chapter 1. This joy is neither conditional nor temporary. *Anandamaya kosha* inspires the intellect sheath (*vijnanamaya*) and calls the other sheaths into existence. Some people best relate to the idea of *anandamaya kosha* as the soul, the spirit, or the universal consciousness. It is the immortal layer of the self.

The Tantric masters used to ask their students: What did you look like before you had a face? Meditating on this question leads to the

YOGA ZONE *YOGA FOR LIFE*

awareness of *anandamaya kosha*. It is indescribable but nonetheless something that can be experienced.

Here is a practice focused on *anandamaya kosha:*

1. Imagine that there is joy at the core of every posture.
2. Feel how every inhale can increase the feeling of joy. Feel how every exhale releases obstacles to bliss.
3. Accept everything that happens in the course of your practice as "ideal."

Exploring the Chakras

NOW FOR A DIFFERENT but parallel idea of the self, a concept that is grounded in the sensory world. The chakras are energy centers in the body that govern the senses. There are seven chakras in all, five of which are tied to the five senses and the five elements (see the chart on pages 100–101).

The sixth chakra is *ajna,* or the third eye, a subtle energy center located in the midbrain area between the eyes. It functions as the command center and the point through which divine inspiration, creativity, and karma (unfinished actions) are initiated. Thoughts can be quieted by focusing on *ajna,* and intuition may be awakened by directing attention to this area.

The seventh chakra, *saraswara,* exists at the very top of the crown of the head. This energy center links us to the universal intelligence that exists all around us.

Each chakra has its own sound *(mantra)* and shape *(yantra).* During meditation, if you chant the *mantra* and visualize the *yantra,* you can maintain the harmony of the chakra. The most important thing is that the chakras remain in balance. Each one controls certain areas of the mind and body; if they are not balanced, certain physical and emotional problems may occur as a result. But by focusing your meditation on the chakras, you can help keep these energy centers in balance and harmony.

The Chakras: Questions for Self-Study

FOCUSING OUR ATTENTION on the chakras also affords us a valuable opportunity for internal reflection and self-study. Perhaps your mind and body have been a bit out of sorts, but you are not quite certain what the trouble is. Here are some questions you can ask yourself to determine which energy centers may need your focus.

MULADHARA
ELEMENT: Earth
PHYSICAL LOCATION OF CHAKRA: Base of the spine
EMOTIONAL AREA GOVERNED: Material needs, survival needs

- Are my actions creating a stable base for me and for those around me, such as company shareholders, clients, fellow employees, immediate family members, friends?
- Do my efforts enable me to provide for my bare necessities, such as housing, food, and clothing?
- Do my actions impinge on the basic security or survival/material needs of others?

The Chakras

CHAKRA	LOCATION OF CHAKRA	ELEMENT	
Muladhara	*Base of the spine*	*Earth*	
Svadisthana	*Sacrum*	*Water*	
Manipura	*Solar plexus*	*Fire*	
Anahata	*Chest*	*Air*	
Vishudda	*Throat*	*Space*	
Ajna, Third Eye	*The forehead, between the eyes*		
Saraswara	*Crown, top of the head*		

EMOTIONAL AREA GOVERNED	SENSE	SOUND (*MANTRA*)	SHAPE (*YANTRA*)
Material things *Survival needs*	*Smell*	LÃM	*Golden square*
Creativity *Likes/Dislikes* *Sexuality*	*Taste*	VÃM	*Silver crescent moon*
Identity *Metabolism* *Healthy Ego* *Extrovert/Introvert qualities*	*Sight*	RÃM	*Two red triangles*
Emotional well-being *Compassion, love, understanding*	*Touch*	YÃM	*Powdery blue star*
Communication with *emotional intelligence*	*Hearing*	HÃM	*White circle*
The command center, the *conductor of the orchestra*		O M	*Gray, egg-* *shaped oval*
Connection to the universe		O M	*Thousand-petaled lotus*

SVADISTHANA

ELEMENT: Water

PHYSICAL LOCATION OF CHAKRA: Sacrum

EMOTIONAL AREA GOVERNED: Creativity, likes/dislikes, sexuality

- Do I like or dislike what I am doing?
- Am I avoiding what I truly dislike?
- Am I acting creatively in my daily life?
- When I create, do I work with others or alone?
- Do I spend my time fantasizing about being somewhere else or doing something else?
- Is there the possibility for more inventiveness, spontaneity, or creativity in my work?

MANIPURA

ELEMENT: Fire

PHYSICAL LOCATION OF CHAKRA: Solar plexus

EMOTIONAL AREA GOVERNED: Identity, ego

- How do my actions define me?
- Are there certain tasks I refuse to do? Why?
- Do I have colleagues who are "higher" or "lower" in status than I am? How does my behavior change when I relate to these different people?
- When I interact with others, do I talk more than I listen?
- Do I use the words *me* and *mine* more often than *us* and *ours*?
- Are my actions strong without being aggressive? Measured without being meager?

ANAHATA

ELEMENT: Air

PHYSICAL LOCATION OF CHAKRA: Chest

EMOTIONAL AREA GOVERNED: Compassion, love, understanding

- Do I care about what I am doing?
- Do I feel compassion and understanding for the people I come in contact with throughout the day?
- Are people's lives enriched by spending time with me?
- Do I really *know* the people I work with? Do I know their names, any shared interests we may have?
- Am I aware of how my actions affect others?

VISHUDDA

ELEMENT: Space

PHYSICAL LOCATION OF CHAKRA: Throat

EMOTIONAL AREA GOVERNED: Communication

- What do my actions communicate to others?
- What do my words communicate to other people?
- What thoughts run through my head during the day?
- Am I comfortable with silence? If not, how do I try to fill it? Am I communicating from fear, ego, or ignorance?
- Do I communicate from my soul?

AJNA, THE THIRD EYE

PHYSICAL LOCATION OF CHAKRA: Forehead between the eyes

EMOTIONAL AREA GOVERNED: Command center

* Are my actions *inspired* or are they *calculated?*
* Do I leave time for moments of "eureka"?
* Do I know everything? Do I walk around in awe?
* Do I control the course of my life? Or am I serving some higher purpose?
* Do I *make* things happen? What would happen if I *let* things happen and went with the flow?

SARASWARA, THE CROWN

PHYSICAL LOCATION OF CHAKRA: Crown of the head

EMOTIONAL AREA GOVERNED: Connection to the universe

* How long has it been since I recognized the divine intelligence within me and all around me?

Recognizing the Divine Within

CLEARLY, THE SELF HAS many facets, and exploring them will take a lifetime. One of the major goals of yoga is to recognize the divine presence within you, and to realize your potential to connect to the higher universal intelligence. The theories behind the *koshas* and the chakras help you to do just that.

Ideally, you will study the concepts in this chapter, let them sink in, and consider them a little more fully every day. Review them often, and find occasion to focus your *asana* practice and your daily meditations on the chakras and the *koshas*. To be sure, it is a journey, but I hope you will continue it for the rest of your life. On this journey you will explore your connection with everything that is, and the inspiration, intuition, and insight of the universe will permeate your life. You will take that experience of unconditional love and joy into every moment of your living, and you will move from the world of *jiva-atman* to the world of *param-atman*. You have undertaken the most important project of your life. Congratulations.

PRANAYAMA

Tuning in to the breath can allow you to withdraw your senses and focus your mind on a single point, which in turn will help you connect with the oneness of the universe. The following breathing exercise, which Swami Venkatesananda used to prescribe, can be done anytime, anywhere. It will sharpen your mind into focus immediately and bring your consciousness back to the union of self and universe that is the goal of yoga.

1. The next time you find yourself feeling overcome or upset or "stuck" in any way, simply exhale completely, then wait.
2. Don't inhale. Wait to see what will happen next. Keep focusing on your body's response, and do not rush through the pause after your exhale. When your body needs to inhale, it will.
3. When an inhale finally comes, notice that your mind has become crystal clear. Do not be surprised if your relationship to whatever concerned you has changed.

Pausing after an exhalation is hardly revolutionary; you do it unconsciously whenever you are preparing the mind to do some extra work. When someone directs your attention to a sound in the distance, you immediately hold your breath ever so slightly to listen. If someone asks you to taste some wonderful food, you place some on your tongue, hold your breath, and savor the food. Finally, if you are going to be injected or pricked with a needle, you very likely hold your breath for a split second as the needle approaches, before it pierces your skin.

Why do we hold our breath in these times of intense concentration? Because the breath stills the mind and enables it to focus its whole attention upon the activity at hand. The body's relaxation response quiets the mind. You can probably think of other examples, and you will probably now notice yourself holding your breath slightly at times when you are trying to concentrate and focus your mind.

Swami Venkatesananda's *pranayama* exercise is a simple one that can be practiced in a few minutes anywhere. A regular and extended practice of paying attention to the breath will enable your consciousness to move away from its preoccupation with the world of duality and instead return you to a state of oneness. Any of the *pranayama* exercises in this book can be used for that purpose. Try to incorporate one or all of them into your daily routine.

ASANA SERIES: FINDING YOUR CORE

From a physical standpoint, the following posture series is important because it taps into your core abdominal muscles and develops strength there, which in turn stabilizes your posture, keeps your spine properly aligned, provides a supple connection between your legs and torso, and protects your back from injury. We all have core abdominal strength to some extent; that strength may, however, be underdeveloped and rarely accessed during normal daily activity.

In the bigger picture, the process of discovering your physical core mirrors the process of finding your spiritual core. As you've seen, there are many ways to seek the spiritual core intellectually. When you combine your physical yoga practice with focused, subtle internal listening, you may be able to unearth inner strength that you only dreamed you could have.

In this posture series both the physical and spiritual cores can be explored simultaneously. The physical act of warming the core, which happens when you stretch your abdominal muscles correctly and mindfully while taking deep, complete breaths, actually encourages the mental relaxation that is necessary for spiritual exploration. As discussed in Chapter 2, when the body is stressed, blood tends to flow to the extremities, away from the core, chilling the body. This practice counteracts that response and sets the stage instead for mindful relaxation and inner discoveries.

The idea of building abdominal strength will not seem new or unusual to anyone who has engaged in an exercise regimen before. Most physical fitness training emphasizes creating powerful abdominal muscles for many of the same reasons I have discussed. What makes the yoga approach different is that these exercises are done with a precision and an awareness that create strength while not sacrificing proper alignment or the ability to breathe freely. You will very likely be surprised at the results. The results of hundreds of mindless abdominal crunches (which interfere with full, complete breathing and correct posture) cannot hold a candle to the benefits—both physical and mental—you can attain from this core strength series.

ASANA SERIES

BREATH WORK

TADAKASANA

BLOWN PALM

VIRABHADRASANA III PREP

BALI SEAL

MOVING LUNGE

INCLINE PLANK

FOREARM PLANK

BALI SEAL

TABLE

PURVOTTANASANA

NAVASANA WITH FOREARMS

NAVASANA WITH KNEES BENT

TARASANA

DANDASANA TWIST

DANDASANA WITH STRAIGHT ARMS

VINYASA DANDASANA FORWARD BEND

VINYASA BRIDGE POSE

SAVASANA

BREATH WORK

Stand tall with your feet separated about a hip width apart. Place your hands on the bony part of your hips; you are touching the front part of your pelvis. Imagine that your pelvis is a basin filled with water. Using your hands, tip the pelvis forward, as if spilling the water out in front of you. Stay in this position and take a few breaths, noticing the sensations that come up in your body. Now tip your pelvis backward, as if spilling the water from the basin behind you. Take a few breaths in this position, and again notice whatever sensations come up in your breathing or in your body.

Now very subtly go back and forth between tipping your pelvis forward and backward, forward and backward, until you arrive at a place where, in your opinion, your pelvis is tipping neither forward nor backward. In this position feel your feet pressing down into the floor and the top of your head moving upward toward the ceiling (lifting from the inside). If your lower rib cage has protruded forward, feel as if your collarbone is lifting up slightly. This should enable your body to find its ideal alignment—an alignment in which your core abdominal strength is activated without interfering with your breathing.

As you inhale, notice your breath moving down toward the base of your spine. As you exhale, begin from below your navel, and as the breath moves out of you, feel the abdominal contraction move upward from your belly toward your solar plexus. Make sure that as you engage those abdominal muscles, you do not disturb the aligned posture that you set up; at the same time do not squeeze those abs. Practice this for several rounds. Notice how breathing with balanced posture is a mini–abdominal workout.

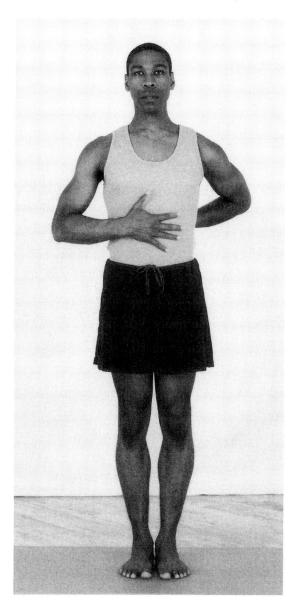

TADAKASANA

Leave your feet a hip width apart, and feel the same connection among your abdominal muscles, legs, and torso. On your inhale raise your arms overhead. On an exhale lower your arms and feel the abdominal contraction initiate just below the navel and move sequentially upward toward the solar plexus. Your shoulder girdle remains positioned directly over your pelvis, which is directly over your heels. On the next inhale, lift your arms into the air and your heels off the floor. On the exhale, lower your arms and heels. Repeat this lifting and lowering process, linked to the inward and outward flow of your breath, three more times. On the fifth lift, stay on the balls of your feet while you exhale and inhale again. Then on the exhale lower your arms and heels. Repeat three more times, lifting on the inhale, staying up for one round of breathing, then lowering on the exhale.

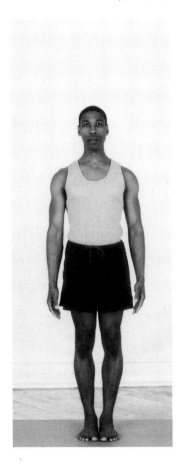

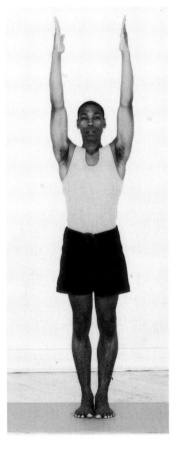

BLOWN PALM

Now experience the strength of the core muscles sustaining you in a side bend. Your feet are flat on the floor, pushing down into the ground. As you inhale, raise your right arm next to your ear, then as you exhale, feel the muscles on the left side of your abdomen and rib cage get shorter, which will allow you to lean to the left. As you inhale, feel the muscles on the right side of your abdomen and rib cage getting longer, stretching open. As you exhale, stay in this position and feel how the abdominal muscles help you maintain a balanced posture front to back. After a couple of breaths, on an inhale stand tall again, and when you exhale, lower the right arm. Before you do the next side, take a moment to observe the effects of your actions.

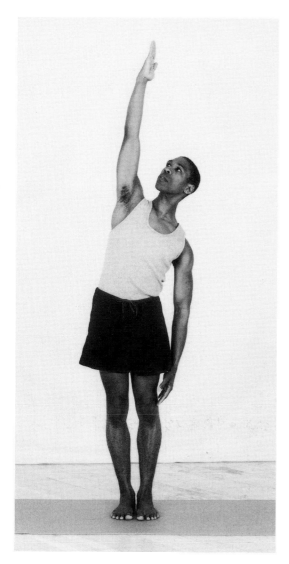

VIRABHADRASANA III PREP

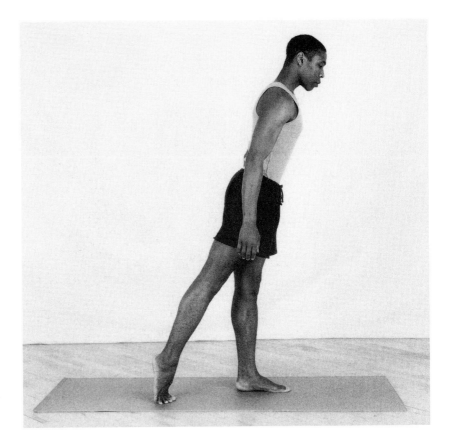

In this position you will use your abdominal muscles to maintain the postural integrity of your torso and pelvis on the front-to-back plane while you are balanced on one leg. Take a step forward with your left foot. Balance on the ball of your right foot. Leaving your arms alongside your hips—or taking them out to the side, if that helps you balance— inhale, and feel a long line running from your right heel through the top of your head; exhale, feeling toned through your abdomen. Inhale, and correct any collapsing of your rib cage over your abdomen; then exhale, correcting any forward or backward tilting of your pelvis. If you are hav- ing difficulty balancing, stay here with your right foot gently touching

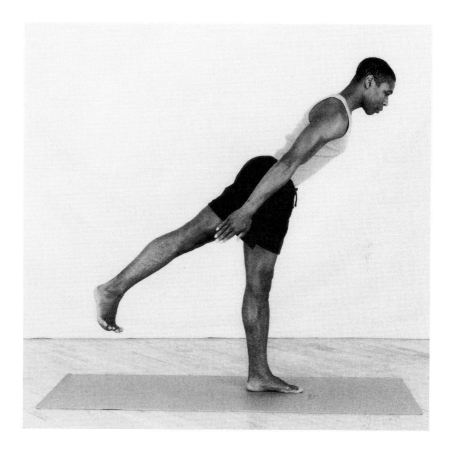

the floor. If you are finding your balance, lift your right foot off the ground, being careful that your right hip does not lift higher than the left. On the inhale check that you are not rounding the spine forward or overarching backward; on the exhale check that you are finding tone in your abdomen and that you are not tilting your pelvis forward or backward. Make sure your standing leg is not locked; keep a slight, slight bend in the knee joint. After staying up for a few breaths, lower yourself on an exhale. Notice the strength and balance you are cultivating. Repeat on the other side.

BALI SEAL

Kneel on the floor. (If this is uncomfortable for your knees or shins, put some padding, such as a pillow or a blanket, underneath; if it is still too uncomfortable, forgo this *asana.*) As you inhale, raise your arms overhead; as you exhale, lower your arms out to the side like wings and slowly lower your seat toward your heels and your belly toward your thighs; stay aware of the abdominal muscles connecting the torso and the legs. As you inhale, feel that you are lengthening forward to come off your thighs (feel the strength required in your abdomen), and as you exhale, try to avoid collapsing your rib cage over your belly. Repeat four to six times.

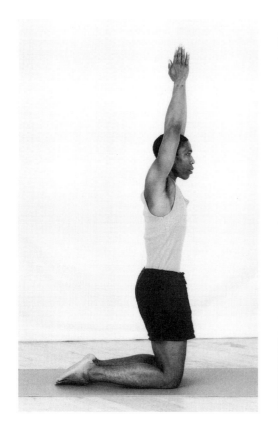

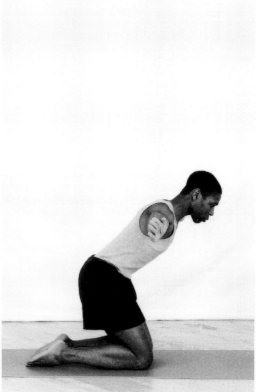

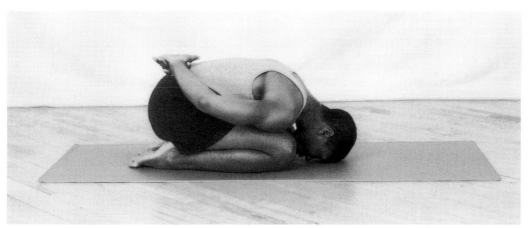

MOVING LUNGE

Come to all fours. Step your left foot forward, and position your left knee directly above your left foot. If you have enough strength in your legs, lift your back (right) knee off the floor and balance on the ball of the right foot; otherwise keep your right knee down. Place your hands on either side of your left foot, and as you inhale, lift your arms out to the sides. Leading with your chest forward, come up to a high lunge with your arms raised overhead. As you exhale, lower your arms to your sides, lower your torso onto your front thigh, and lower your hands to either side of your left foot. On the inhale rise up again. Make sure that you are not leading with your chin, which would put pressure on the back of your neck. On the exhale, lower yourself, taking care to keep your chin down—in fact, relax your head and neck on the way down. As you practice this Moving Lunge sequence, observe that you are not collapsing your chest over your belly as you exhale and that you are not relying on your shoulders to lift you up as you inhale. Observe that the strength in your abdomen and back is keeping you strong and centered.

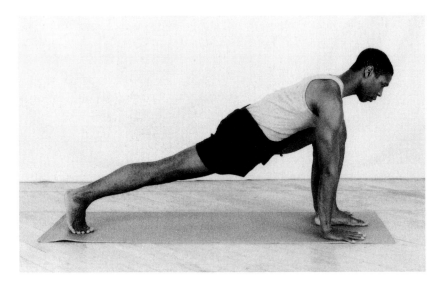

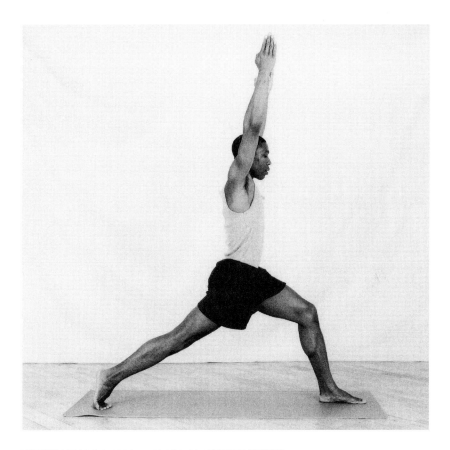

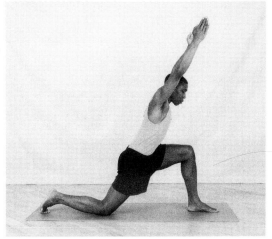

INCLINE PLANK

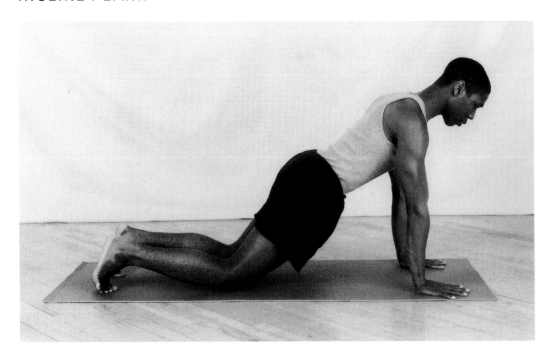

Practice this position first on your knees, then as a full plank. Start again on all fours. Walk your knees backward about a foot or so. Keep your hands more or less underneath your shoulders. Discover the place where your abdominal muscles are engaged and support you, and where your seat is not rising up into the air and your pelvis is not dropping downward. In this place you can feel an extension from the base of your spine out through the top of your head. Your arms are supporting some of your weight, but you are not pushing yourself away from the floor; your shoulder blades should be moving down your back and closer together but not so close that they are squeezing. Hold this posture, and on the inhale breathe down the spine; on the exhale breathe up the spine.

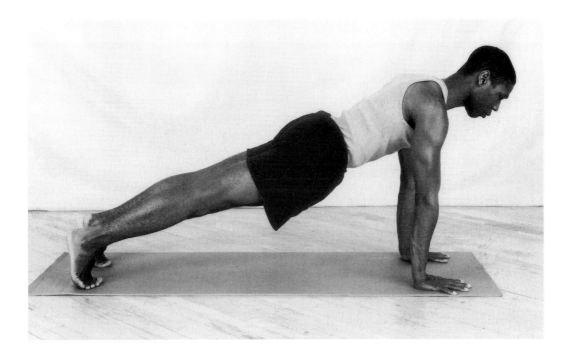

If you can comfortably maintain this posture for six breaths, try lifting your knees off the floor for Incline Plank position. In this posture you resemble a board placed at an incline, from your heels to the top of your head. Stay in this position for six to eight breaths.

FOREARM PLANK

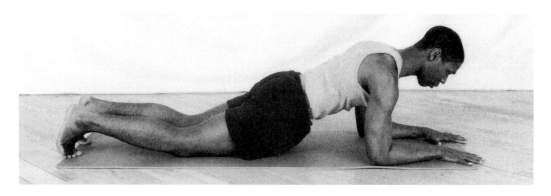

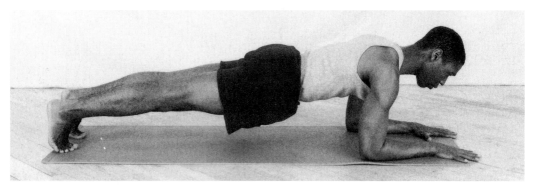

Forearm Plank is similar to Incline Plank. The difference is that Forearm Plank has a wider base; instead of the palms alone, the elbows, forearms, and palms provide the base. You may think this pose is easier than Incline Plank; for many it is as challenging, if not more so. Begin on all fours, as you did for Incline Plank, but now drop your forearms down onto the floor so that your elbows are underneath your shoulders. Practice this pose with your knees on the floor if you need to; eventually your knees will come off the ground, and you will create a straight line from your heels to the back of your head. As you inhale and exhale, take long, smooth breaths.

The breathing reminds you of the core strength that is required and developed in this posture! After six to eight breaths you are ready to rest.

BALI SEAL

After the challenging plank postures, practice Bali Seal (see page 116) to rest. Take the awareness of your core strength that you have been developing into this posture. Observe if you have heightened your ability to maintain your aligned posture through this pose since beginning the practice.

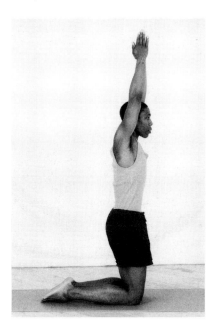
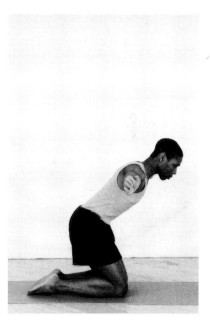

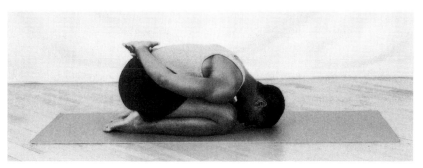

TABLE

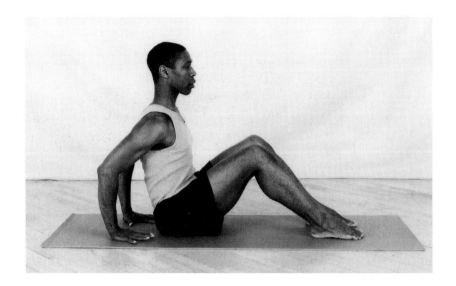

After having practiced Bali Seal, sit up, and place your hands on the floor behind you. Figure out what the best place is for your hands; you may prefer them to be wider than your shoulders or closer to your hips, depending on the flexibility of your wrists. Place your feet on the floor about two feet away from your hips (or thereabouts). As you inhale, feel your rib cage broaden and lift away from your pelvis. As you exhale, feel your lower belly contract, creating stability in your pelvis (so it does not move either forward or backward and put pressure on the lower back).

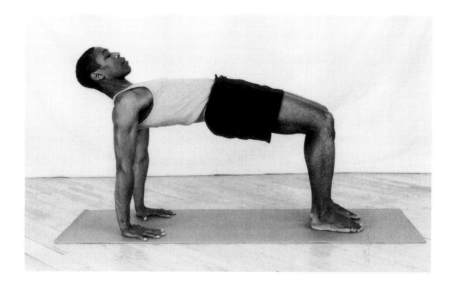

On your next inhale, lift your hips off the floor, and imagine bringing your pelvis forward toward your knees. Be careful that you are not push-ing down on your hands to lift your hips up off the floor. On the exhale remain in the air. Use the core strength in your back, abdomen, and legs to create this four-legged table. Remain for four to eight breaths.

PURVOTTANASANA

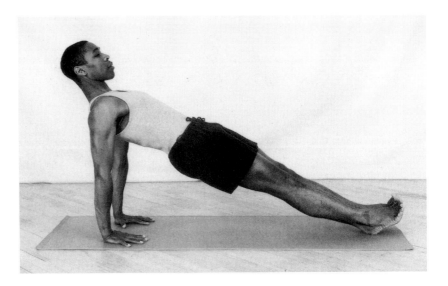

If your wrists are bothering you after Table, you may consider skipping *Purvottanasana* until you develop the core strength for this pose. Moving into this posture from Table is actually an effective transition. From Table, extend your right leg forward onto the floor. Don't let your hips drop! Next extend your left leg. Breathe into your chest, and feel the spine in the upper part of your back drawing into your body. Exhale, feeling the strength in your legs and abdomen.

NAVASANA

Begin with your pelvis balanced on your sitting bones so that your spine is held tall. Bend your knees and place your toes on the floor. Let your hands support behind your knees. On the inhale breathe into the top corners of your chest. On the exhale contract the muscles in your abdomen and lift your legs up off the floor with knees bent, then straighten them. It does not matter how high you lift. Inhale, coming to balance on your sitting bones. Do not sink into your lower back; in fact, draw your ribcage away from your hip structure. You may choose to extend your arms in front of you, parallel to the floor. On the exhale, bend your knees and lower your feet onto the floor. Repeat this sequence two more times.

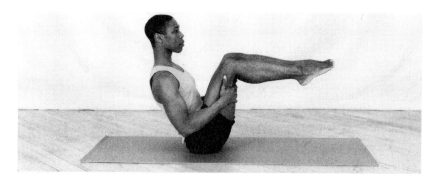

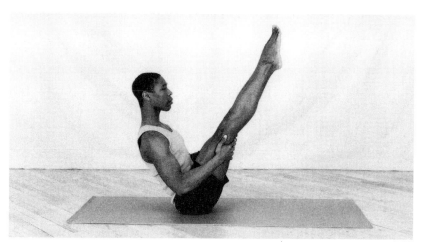

NAVASANA VARIATION

If you found *Navasana* too challenging, start with this position and develop into it over time. Begin the same way, with your pelvis balanced on your sitting bones so that your spine is held tall and your knees bent with your toes on the floor. Lower your forearms onto the floor behind you, so that you are able to support your torso without putting any strain on your shoulder girdle. Inhale and fill the top corners of your chest. Exhale and, as you lift your toes off the floor, draw in your abdominal muscles (starting from below the navel and working up toward the solar plexus). Keep your shins parallel to the floor. Do not worry how high your legs go; keep your knees bent and your spine tall. Inhale again, and on the exhale lower your feet to the floor. Practice this sequence two more times.

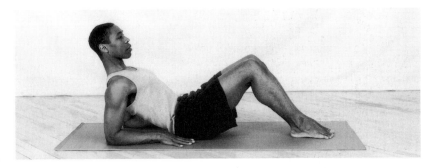

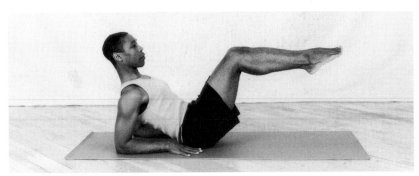

TARASANA

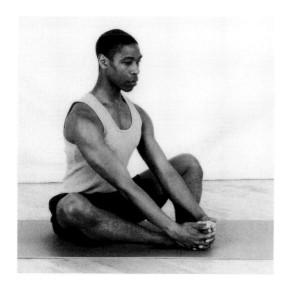 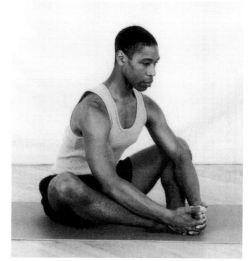

After doing the *Navasana* variations, it is important to stretch the back of your body. While you are still sitting on the floor, let your knees drop open, and let the soles of your feet touch each other. Grab onto your shins or ankles, and fold your torso over your outstretched legs. You may get a better stretch through the whole of your back if your heels are farther away from you. After releasing the back, reach your torso forward and lift it upward.

DANDASANA TWIST

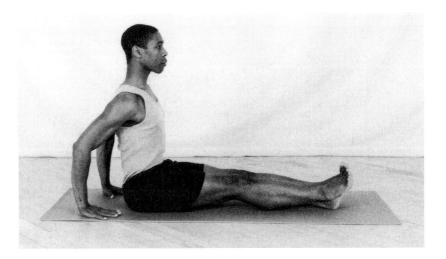

Sitting with your legs straight out in front of you, check again that your pelvis is not tipping backward, which would put a strain on your lower back or cause you to exaggerate the use of your upper back. Bend your right leg, and place your right foot on the outside of your left knee. Hug your right knee with your left arm. Inhale, and feel an extension out through the top crown of your head.

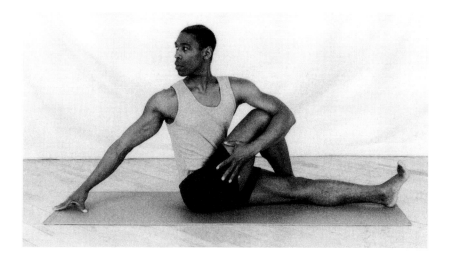

Exhale, and use your abdominal muscles to initiate a twist to look back over your right shoulder. With every inhale draw yourself up a little taller; with every exhale rotate from the abdomen. Try not to use your arms to motor you into the Twist; they can provide supplementary strength, but let your abdominal muscles be the major twisting force. Repeat on the other side.

DANDASANA WITH STRAIGHT ARMS

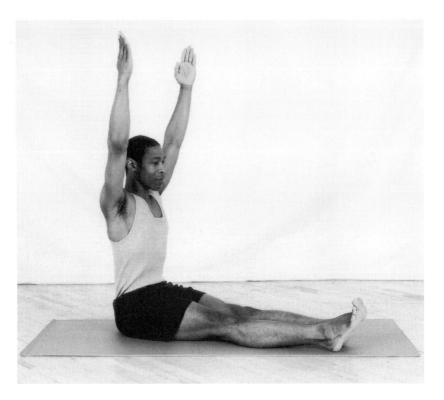

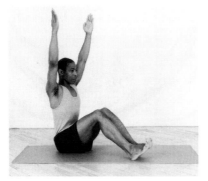

In this version of *Dandasana,* you are going to raise your arms straight up into the air. The tendency will be to either put tension into the shoulders or to lose the strength and connection you have been developing with your core muscles (the abdominals, legs, and back). Be liberal about bending your knees so that you do not rock backward. On the inhale feel your rib cage lifting away from your pelvis, and on the exhale notice the strength at your core. Repeat for six cycles of inhale and exhale.

VINYASA DANDASANA FORWARD BEND

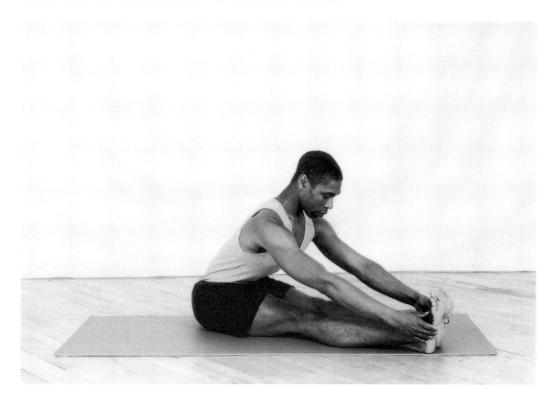

Start at *Dandasana* with Straight Arms. On an exhale extend your torso out over your legs. (Notice the stretching along each vertebra.) On an inhale reach your chest forward as you raise your arms and torso back up again. Repeat three more times. On the way down and on the way up take your time to feel the stretching of the back of your body, then the stretching of the front of your body, respectively.

VINYASA BRIDGE POSE

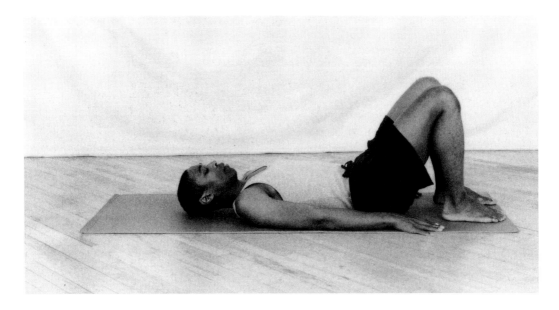

Lie down on your back, but keep your knees bent and your feet flat on the floor. Lift your shoulders up toward your ears, ever so slightly.

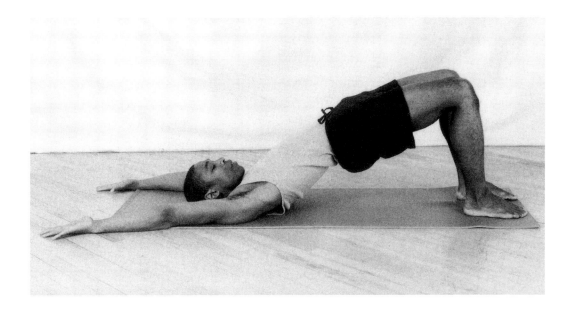

As you inhale, lift your pelvis off the floor while pressing your feet down into the ground. You may reach your arms overhead and extend them to the floor behind you, as shown, or keep them alongside your body. As you exhale, lower your pelvis to the floor, starting with your upper back, then your middle back, and lastly your lower back, as you lower your arms to the floor. Use long, smooth breaths. Inhale, raising the hips; exhale, lowering one vertebra at a time. Repeat for six cycles of inhale and exhale.

SAVASANA

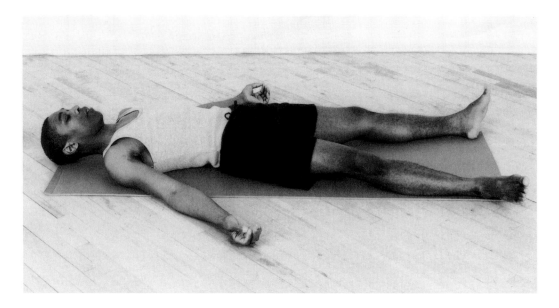

As you lie on the floor, extend your legs, letting your feet drop open. Draw your shoulder blades closer together and down your back so that your chest feels open and relaxed. Gently move your head from side to side until you find a comfortable resting position. Close your eyes, and observe your breathing without changing it. Try not to interfere with the inhalation or exhalation; try not to disturb the pauses in between. Stay alert, but let go of the need to do anything. Remain here for as long as you like (but at least five minutes).

VARIATIONS ON THIS *ASANA* SERIES

Before you begin your physical practice, quiet your mind with the practice of *pranayama.* Try *ujjayi pranayama* (see page 36), Alternate Nostril Breathing (see page 151), or the *Kriya* Yoga Breath (see page 153).

Pick a *kosha* (see page 93), and focus your *asana* practice upon it.

Follow this *asana* practice with a meditation on the chakras (see page 98), to create balance among them. Meditate for a few minutes on the *mantra* (sound) and *yantra* (shape) that correspond to each of the seven chakras. Or if you prefer, pick one chakra, and focus your attention solely on its *mantra* and *yantra.*

A MEDITATION ON YOUR NAME

You may not realize what a powerful hold your name has on you. Have you ever been walking through a noisy public place and heard your name, or thought you did? Chances are you felt a strong urge to stop and seek the source. You have probably heard or seen your name thousands upon thousands of times by now. But what does that name really have to do with *you* and your deeper self? We are all familiar with the Shakespeare quotation "A rose by any other name would smell as sweet," but do we really feel comfortable disassociating ourselves from our given names?

In a yoga context, your name can be turned into a *mantra*, or tool for the mind, that can help you transcend outmoded ideas of who you are. In the following meditation you will draw your attention to the associations that you have attached to your name. Before you begin the exercise, read through the instructions to make sure you understand them completely. Practice the meditation with your eyes closed; opening and closing your eyes to read the next step would be distracting.

1. Sit comfortably in a position that you can maintain for ten to fifteen minutes. A cross-legged seat may be appropriate for some; for others sitting upright in a chair will create greater ease and stability.
2. Cross your arms over your chest so that your right hand is touching the left side of your rib cage and your left hand is touching the right side of your rib cage.
3. Close your eyes, and feel the expansion and contraction of your rib cage. After a while, if you detect that one side of your chest is expanding more than the other, adjust your arms so that the arm

that was on the bottom now crosses over on top of the other arm. This will adjust the pressure on the side that is expanding more.

4. When both sides of your rib cage are expanding equally, lower your hands, allowing the backs of the hands to rest on top of your knees or thighs.

5. Imagine that you are walking through a forest, a dense wooded forest. Climb over any fallen logs in your path, and part any branches that obstruct your way. Keep walking. Arrive at a clearing, an open area that is circular in shape, surrounded on all sides by the forest.

6. Stand in the middle of the clearing, and silently call out your name. If possible, choose a nickname that is one or two syllables. If a multisyllabic variation means more to you, however, use it.

7. Every time you call out your name, let a different aspect of your personality emerge from the forest (e.g., the sad you, the strong you, the manipulative you, the loving you).

8. Repeat, bringing forth as many aspects of yourself as you can muster.

9. With one last silent yell, call out your name and feel all these personalities merge together simultaneously. Feel that collective identity. Experience yourself as you were before you were given a name.

10. Remain still with that experience for five to ten minutes, then reground your energy by bringing your palms over your face and gently guiding the energy down your face, throat, neck, chest, solar plexus, and navel and into your legs.

11. Bring your awareness of who you really are with you into the rest of your day.

5

FINDING BALANCE

Memory and impression have similar forms.
They give birth to our tendencies, which operate continuously
to shape our lives, even if their cause is separated from
their effect by time, by place, or by lifetimes.

PATANJALI, *YOGA SUTRAS*, CHAPTER 4, VERSE 7

S YOU'VE SEEN, ONE OF THE REMARKABLE EFFECTS OF A BALANCED PHYSICAL YOGA PRACTICE IS A SENSE OF CONTROL OVER YOUR BODY, YOUR MIND, AND ULTIMATELY—USING THAT PHYSICAL AND MENTAL discipline—your own destiny. The law of karma, one of the central parts of any lifelong yoga practice, states that every action you make, no matter how small, has an effect that will return to you at some point. Thus, by exerting control over your actions and recognizing your tendencies toward good and bad, you can ultimately control your own future. Karma is a cycle of cause and effect that, once understood, will give you a framework to understand Yoga for Life.

The actions I am talking about may be small or very large. Whether you are in a grocery store, at your place of employment, at home with your family, or on vacation in the tropics, you are always subject to the law of cause and effect. Each one of your actions, positive or negative, will return to you at some point; but if you are mindful of the actions you take, you will have control over their effects. This karmic cycle will affect you until you die and perhaps even in lives still to come. The yoga writings tell us that there are three types of karma: *sanctita karma,* which is the accumulation of karma from past lives; *prarabhda karma,* which is the accumulation of unfinished actions you are currently dealing with in this life; and *agami-karma,* the incomplete actions from this lifetime that you will ultimately finish in the future, in this lifetime or the next. We have a lot of work waiting for us.

The ancient yogis believed that we experience multiple lives. You do not have to believe this if you prefer, but it is still wise to pay attention to the law of karma as it relates to your actions in this lifetime. Even if you reject the notion of past and future lives, realize that your actions are shaping your destiny in this life. If, on the other hand, you are especially enthusiastic about the concept of other lives, take care not to get bogged down in wondering who you were or will be. We really do not and cannot know; our brains can barely handle the information of this life, let alone figure out what happened in lifetimes past. When we dwell on the past and the future, we blind ourselves to the present moment.

The Karmic Cycle

HOW THEN DOES KARMA OPERATE? If all our actions, positive and negative, will eventually return to us, how does that work? When an action remains incomplete—when it has not been rectified, made right, or amended, when it has not come full circle—it does not simply disappear into a void somewhere. Say, in the most obvious example, you kick a dog and feel bad about it for a while but soon forget it ever happened. The universe has made a record of your action and intention, called a *samskara,* and that *samskara* lodges itself deep in your consciousness. You will eventually come back to this action in the future, even if you have momentarily erased it from the forefront of your memory. You will complete the unfinished action. You have the free will to procrastinate as much as you want, but at the end of the day, the leftover chores will still be waiting for you. If you subscribe to the idea of future lives, yoga theory holds that you will get some time off after you die, as a child gets a summer vacation, and if you have more studies to finish, you will come back for the next grade. If your studies are complete, you will remain in the state of bliss.

No straightforward logic applies to the release of *samskaras* (those individual karmic lessons). In the case of the kicked dog, you will probably not get the opportunity to meet that dog in another incarnation, or even a few years down the road in this lifetime, and apologize for your short temper. But the *samskara* created by your action will lodge in *annomaya, pranamaya, manomaya,* and *vijnanamaya koshas* (see Chapter 4). Your body and your consciousness are virtual storehouses for your unfinished actions.

The *samskaras* are like imprints left on your consciousness by habitual actions. They are the grooves that are very difficult to avoid falling into again and again. They are a well-traveled road that leads nowhere. As a result, our thoughtless actions will tend toward habits and patterns that we have acted out in the past. The way to break this cycle is to deal with the unfinished actions. Karma, like a spiritual "to do" list, is stored in six of the seven chakras. (The seventh, the one located at the crown of the head, does not store karma.) All you must do is access that "to do" list with a thoughtful yoga practice and a deepening understanding of your own soul and its habits and tendencies. In fact, whole branches of yoga are devoted to doing this; *karma yoga* (selfless service) and *bhakti yoga* (devotional yoga) believe that when we perform actions that are dedicated to the benefit of others or to glorifying God, we are purifying our own consciousness and letting go of our own egos.

When you are engaged in life on the dual plane (where the mind, ego, and body dominate), your karma will not be released all at once. Imagine how overwhelming that would be! Instead, you are given your lessons in manageable bits and pieces. The situations you find yourself in do not arise by accident; they are programmed especially for you. If you consciously, or unconsciously through lack of awareness, ignore the opportunity to resolve a particular *samskara,* that individual lesson will linger until, like a towering pile of dirty laundry, you can no longer avoid putting it off.

Dharma: A Path Through Life's Challenges

IN ORDER TO HELP us work through our karma, our unfinished lessons, as efficiently as possible, the universe has set us up with a dharma, a path that, if we follow it, will keep us from getting bogged down in the daily grind.

Your dharma is set up at the moment of your conception. According to the yoga teachings, during the act of lovemaking the mixing of masculine and feminine energies sets up a unique magnetic vibration that draws out from the ocean of unbound energy a "drop" of consciousness that enters into the couple's orbit. When the sperm and egg meet, the drop of consciousness (the soul) initiates life. The cells begin splitting, from one to two, two to four, four to sixteen, and so on at a rate unique to that being—the pulse of that splitting is called *nadi,* the pulse of life. The soul is said to be attracted to a particular couple because their personalities, financial circumstances, values, and virtues are such that they will enable the child to accelerate through his or her unfinished actions and recognize that his or her ultimate reality is not determined by this dual world.

Now *anandamaya kosha,* or soul, is very clear about what its dharma is, but unfortunately, as we discovered in Chapter 4, the four layers on top of that *kosha* can obstruct our ability to recognize our true path in life. Instead of letting the soul lead the way, the mind, ego, and emotions will engage in some backseat driving, often steering us off our true path.

That is not to say that there is only one path you must take, and if you miss it, all is lost. Although one overriding dharma leads you through life, there are also minipaths along the way. One's dharma is not strictly one's career, for example; a man might have a dharma as an office worker, a father, a husband, a son, a member of the Chamber of Commerce, and so forth. Each of these roles involves expectations specific to the individual. All fathers, all husbands, all sons are not the same because although the roles are similar, the specific details of the situations from person to person can be quite different, and those specific situations have been custom-designed for your individual needs. In each of your various roles you have an opportunity to encounter, observe, and improve different aspects of your personality.

Taking a closer look at the various roles you play throughout the day, and how you act in them, may start to give you an understanding of the overriding role that you are here to play. You may discover that you are on target, engaged in activities and associations that are most helpful to your personal growth and development. Or you may discover that you have strayed from the path, the dharma, that you should be following. If you have slipped, your yoga practice can help you find your way back onto the path, and enable you to most efficiently work through the lessons you still have to finish.

Career Karma and Dharma

YOU ARE NOT YOUR JOB, but if you became so wrapped up in work that you deluded yourself into thinking that what you do for a living is the sum total of your identity, you would not be the first person to do so. In the same way, many of us can become so immersed in our hobbies and pleasures that we define ourselves only by what we do in our spare time. You are neither your labors nor your pleasures, but each of these things can be a mirror for you to examine who you really are.

Our purpose in being here, after all, is to remember who we really are—unbound by time and form—and to make sure that the major parts of the day are filled with activities that will help us remain focused on our purpose. In that sense, the things we do both at work and at play can provide us with valuable opportunities to finish up those unfinished lessons (*samskaras*).

If you, like the average person in the United States, work forty hours a week, from a time management perspective alone it would help if you approached your career as an opportunity to work out karma and help others work out theirs. Your dharma has set you up with certain skills that you may apply however and wherever you choose.

So consider why you will go to work tomorrow. If you are retired or not working, consider how you will use your spare time. What purpose will you fulfill? At the end of the day, will you feel rejuvenated and energized, as you do at the end of a good yoga practice? If not, why? What changes could you make to your job in order to make it a more transformational experience? Given that you are here on Earth to work out the unfinished lessons lodged in your chakras, perhaps those are the notes you should be making in your Palm Pilot!

In the *Bhagavad Gita*, Arjuna's "job" was to go to war, to be in combat against members of his own family. In the book, which is one of the most important texts of yoga, Arjuna learns a soul-inspired way to do his very difficult job. If you think it is impossible to perform your own job or go about your day in a way that enables you to work out your karma, think again.

Ten Ego-Reducing Actions

OUR EGO TENDS TO BE the biggest barrier in the way of accepting the dharma that has been created for us and the karma stored in our chakras. When your only concern is for yourself, you are prioritizing your experience over that of the world around you. But the universe is far too complex to center on the desires of any one individual, and when you let your ego guide your path, you miss many opportunities.

Here are ten actions (called *yamas* and *niyamas*) that will help you transcend your ego and become more accepting of whatever the universe has in store for you, your dharma. The five *yamas*—nonviolence or noninjury, truthfulness, nonstealing, nonhoarding, and moving with God—suggest how you should orient yourself in order to be one with the natural flow of the universe. The five *niyamas*—purity, contentment, self-discipline, self-study, and acting with devotion—suggest the spirit in which we should act. To use the analogy of surfing, the *yamas* teach us how to position our board in the path of the waves, while the *niyamas* point out the style in which to stay up and enjoy the ride to the fullest extent.

THE *YAMAS*

By practicing nonviolence or noninjury *(ahimsa)*, you are making sure that your thoughts, words, and actions are always helping and not harming yourself and those around you. The intention of the universe is not to punish, it is to help everyone achieve the lessons they need to achieve.

The second *yama* is truthfulness, or *satya.* When your consciousness is clear, there is only truth. Lying may boost your status in the material world, in this plane of consciousness, but it will not help you achieve the ultimate goals the universe has in store for you.

Nonstealing, or *asteya,* aligns you with the flow of the universe. All the reasons you may have to steal from others stem from a perceived deficiency, but deficiencies are always illusions. The universe has already given you everything you need. You have no need to steal when everything you need is already yours.

Nonhoarding, or *aparigraha*, is another key *yama*. When you hoard material goods, ideas, or even friends, you are making the judgment that the universe will not continue to provide you with everything you need. You are putting too much stock in the material world and not enough faith in the higher universe. By hoarding, you not only interfere with your own ability to acquire new experiences, you also interfere with the ability of those around you to benefit from what the universe has created.

Moving with God, or *bramacharya*, refers to merging our own divine energy with the divine energy all around us. Recognize the divinity within you and seek to use your divine energy as God would use it. This is the union that is at the heart of yoga.

THE *NIYAMAS*

Once you have oriented yourself to be in the natural flow of the universe, you want to do your best to remain in its path. If there is purity, or *saucha*, to your actions, you are acting in synchronicity with the nature of the universe. When your body is full of stress and tension and your mind is filled with fantasies and selfish thoughts, you obscure the purity at your core. Pure actions emanate from a clean body and a pure mind.

The second *niyama*, contentment or *santosha*, is to be expected once you give yourself over to the natural flow. You are a product of the universe and not vice versa. When you do not challenge the universe's intentions for you, you find yourself content and in harmony.

Self-discipline, or *tapas*, is a *niyama* that has been a theme throughout this book. With self-discipline you can focus your attention, perfect the *asana* positions, and control your breathing. You can control your thoughts and actions in order to confront life's unfinished lessons and remain on the path the universe has set for you. You will avoid the fleeting desires of the material world and instead focus on what brings about true happiness—the divinity within you and all around you.

Self-study, or *svadyaya*, makes people unique from all other life-forms. Applying self-study to your actions prevents you from repeating habits and patterns (those *samskaras* again). With self-study you can also free yourself from limits and boundaries. Studying spiritual texts and applying them to your own life is a form of *svadyaya*.

Acting with devotion, or *isvara pranidhana*, is one of the highest forms of ego-nullification. If you dedicate each and every action to the universe, in gratitude for your presence here, everything you do is for a higher purpose. This selflessness in action will help expose you to the inspiration and insight all around you.

All of the *yamas* and *niyamas* boil down to one single concept: we have been put here in order to love. The foundation of the universe is unconditional love—it is made of harmony and nonconflict. When we act in accordance with the universe, there is only love, and there is so much possibility.

ALTERNATE NOSTRIL BREATHING

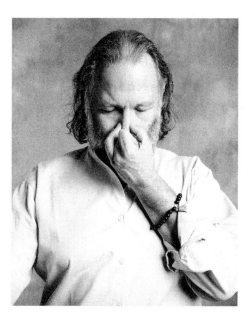

Many breathing techniques can be used to create balance, but one of the most powerful is Alternate Nostril Breathing. Did you know that during the course of the day, one nostril is always more dominant, more open to inhaling and exhaling, than the other? In general, every eighty-eight minutes one side is dominant, then for two minutes they are equally open, and then dominance switches to the other side. You may have noticed this phenomenon most obviously when you have had a cold—one nostril is often stuffed up and then magically clears; then the other side becomes congested.

The practice of Alternate Nostril Breathing leads to the balanced flow of *prana* (energy) and oxygen through both nostrils and sets up a state of balance throughout the nervous system. That is because as the nostrils switch their dominance from right to left, so too do the hemispheres of the brain.

In yoga, dominance of the breath in the right nostril is associated with activity, heat, and the left side of the brain. Dominance of the breath in the left nostril is associated with cooling, calmness, and the right side of the brain. After you practice Alternate Nostril Breathing, the flow of breath through both nostrils is neutralized and your energy flows through a central, balanced channel of consciousness. Here's how you do it:

1. Take a comfortable seated position, holding your spine tall.
2. Drop your chin down toward your chest in a way that allows your neck to remain long. Do not round your shoulders forward or lift your shoulder girdle off your rib cage. When done properly, this "chin-lock," called *jalandara-bandha,* should not create tension in your neck or throat.
3. Open your right palm. Bend your first two fingers down into the palm. The thumb, ring finger, and pinky finger should remain upright. This hand position is called Vishnu Mudra.
4. Raise your right hand so that the thumb blocks your right nostril and the ring finger blocks your left nostril. Place the thumb and ring finger on pressure points just below the hard cartilage in the nose. Pressing on these points affects the *prana's* ability to move to the left side or the right.
5. Close your eyes.
6. Inhale through your right nostril by gently sliding your thumb alongside the right nostril—while keeping your left nostril blocked.
7. Block both nostrils, and pause for a few seconds.
8. Exhale through your left nostril—make space by sliding your ring finger alongside the nostril. Keep your right nostril blocked.

9. Inhale through your left nostril (the same side you just exhaled from).

10. Block both nostrils and pause for a few seconds.

11. Exhale through your right nostril.

12. This completes one round of Alternate Nostril Breathing. On most days you will need to practice multiple rounds before you can bring both nostrils, both sides of the brain, and the left and right energy channels into balance.

13. Once you feel that equilibrium has been established, keep your eyes closed, but lower your right hand from your nostrils. Remain in this quiet, balanced, and contemplative state for a few minutes.

PARAMAHANSA YOGANANDA'S *KRIYA* YOGA BREATH

Another powerful breathing technique that can be used either as a follow-up to Alternate Nostril Breathing or as a substitute for it is Paramahansa Yogananda's *Kriya* Yoga Breath. Yogananda initiated Mani Finger into this particular breathing technique. It isolates the energy in the central channel and is designed to accelerate the karmic cycle. Doing a single round of this technique with complete passion and sincerity is said to bring the practitioner a year closer to immersion in the soul consciousness. Here is how to do it:

1. In a seated position, holding your spine tall and your eyes closed, bring your awareness to the central cord of consciousness running down through the center of your torso.

2. Bring your attention to the base of your spine. Take a few moments, and isolate your awareness in that area.

3. To the extent that you are still aware of your breathing, bring your attention to your inhalation. Follow that inhalation upward from the base of the spine toward the top of your head.

4. On your exhalation, follow your breath down the spine until your attention reaches the base of the spine again.

5. This completes one round.

6. Practice additional rounds, and really absorb your attention into what you are doing. It may help to add a visualization of light traveling up and down your spine (if you are visually inclined) or to link the sounds of *hum* to the inhalation and *sah* to the exhalation (if you are aurally inclined). Linking light or sound to your awareness of energy movement will deepen your experience of this technique.

   At a certain point your desire to follow the energy up and down your spine will stop, and allow your attention to focus on the point between your eyebrows and in the center of the brain. This point, called *ajna,* is the command center, the point where karma is conducted into being. This meditation/breathing technique should, as a result, help you be more clear about how to resolve whatever difficulties are facing you.

6

RESTORING THE BODY

The practice of yoga will be firmly rooted
when it is maintained consistently and with
dedication over a long period.

PATANJALI, *YOGA SUTRAS*, CHAPTER I, VERSE 14

YOU MAY HAVE HEARD OF A BRANCH OF YOGA CALLED RESTORATIVE YOGA, IN WHICH YOU HOLD POSTURES FOR EVER LONGER PERIODS OF TIME, FOCUSING ON ALIGNMENT AND THE HEALING BENEFITS THAT YOGA POSTURES CAN HAVE on the body. Restorative yoga is a wonderful way to let the body rejuvenate and heal itself, and it is also a fantastic way to practice *vairagya* (dispassion, or nonconcern for results). In fact, the more you can learn to let go, the more rewarding your experience will be.

Restorative yoga can be used to help treat certain ailments; it may also be practiced by people with physical limitations or injuries. If you are encumbered by physical problems you may be surprised to discover that such a simple focus on alignment and relaxation can do so much to improve existing injuries and chronic pain. One word of caution, however: as therapeutic as these positions may be, it is still possible to injure yourself if you do them incorrectly. Please consult your doctor before beginning any new exercise regimen, particularly if you have injuries or other physical difficulties.

The first thing you will notice about the restorative yoga sequence that follows—or any restorative yoga class—is that the postures are held for longer periods of time, often ten to fifteen minutes or more. This gives the body time to relax, rejuvenate, and fully absorb all the healing benefits of each pose. For an example, consider the Viparita Karani pose (see page 163). This is an inverted pose, meaning the body is in the opposite alignment than it would be in normal daily life, with the legs above the head. By doing this simple inversion, you redirect the blood flow in the body and remove some of the pressure that builds up in the legs and feet. This simple reversal can be powerfully rejuvenating.

Another distinguishing characteristic of restorative yoga is the use of props. In the positions that follow you will use folded blankets, foam blocks, and straps in order to put your body into the correct alignment with minimal effort. The props also minimize strain and ensure that the body is fully supported. Once you begin using these aids you will not be able to imagine your restorative practice without them.

The physical benefits of restorative yoga aside, you will also find that moving into a state of complete relaxation provides you with the opportunity to quiet your mind completely. Gone are all hopes and expectations, the breeding ground for frustration. You are primed for acceptance, for self-study, and for all of the awakenings that come along with it.

The following sequence will induce your brain waves to change from their waking beta rhythm to a slower-moving alpha rhythm. The first couple of times you practice this sequence, you may nod off. That's okay. Eventually you will be able to remain alert in your sleep— your mind will retire to the background, but you will enter the state of *yoga nidra,* the sleepless sleep, where you will be awake to the body surrendering itself to the healing powers of *samadhi.*

Above all, restorative yoga is gentle, relaxing, and deeply meditative. The emphasis in the sequence that follows, as in any yoga practice, is not on performance. Try to make these positions effortless, and remain as unconcerned as possible with the results. Focus on your breath and quiet your mind. It may be difficult to let go at first, but you will find that as you practice the sequence, both physical and mental stress dissipate, leaving you refreshed and renewed. Even when practicing the other *asana* series in this book, you may wish to end each practice with one or two of these restorative poses.

A RESTORATIVE YOGA SERIES

You will need a thick blanket, an eye bag (scented or unscented), two large firm pillows or a yoga bolster, and a belt.

ASANA SERIES

BACK ARCH/HEART OPENER

SUPPORTED CHILD'S POSE

VIPARITA KARANI

SUPPORTED *SAVASANA*

BACK ARCH/HEART OPENER *(10 minutes)*

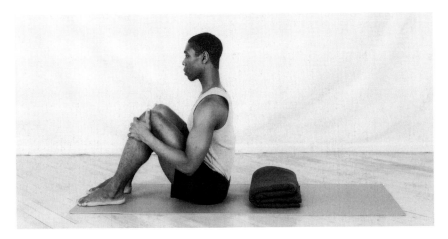

Take the blanket, and fold it into a rectangular shape—if your back is more flexible, you will want to fold your blanket more thickly. Place the blanket on the floor, then lie down on top of it so that your head is just off the blanket and it supports your upper back without putting strain on your lower back.

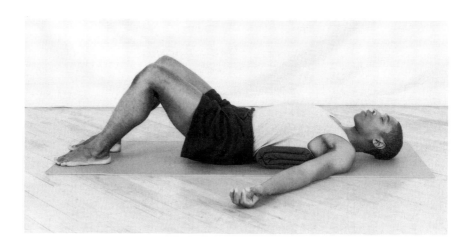

Depending on the original alignment of your neck and head, you may
need some support underneath your head as well. Let your arms extend
out to your sides. Cover your eyes with the eye pillow. Extend your legs
onto the floor, or keep them bent. Set a timer for ten minutes. If your timer
has a loud buzz or ring to it, you may choose instead to play a piece of
music that lasts about ten minutes.

To come out of this position, bend your knees into your chest and gently
roll over to your right side to come off the blanket.

SUPPORTED CHILD'S POSE *(5 minutes)*

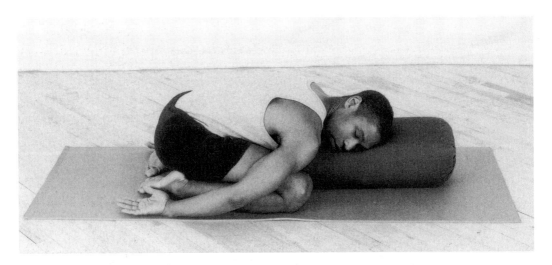

Kneel on the floor with your knees wide enough apart that the pillows or bolster can come in between. Lower your belly down on the pillows/bolster, and give your weight over to it. Turn your head to one side or the other. Halfway through, switch your head to the other side so your neck remains balanced.

VIPARITA KARANI (5 minutes)

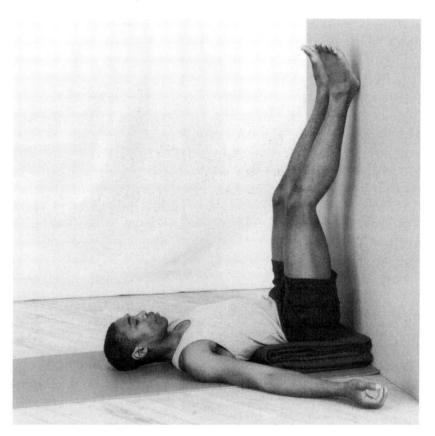

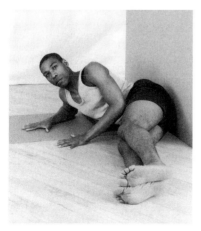

This is a wonderful restorative position. Find some open wall space where you are practicing. Lie down on the floor, and take your legs up the wall in such a way that your lower back stays down on the floor, or on a blanket or bolster. You may need to bend your knees; although your legs will get a stretch in this pose, the reason for coming into it is not for the stretch. Use the eye pillow to cover your eyes and relax their muscles and the rest of the face. Let the ground support you. Let your breathing adjust to this position.

SUPPORTED *SAVASANA (15 minutes)*

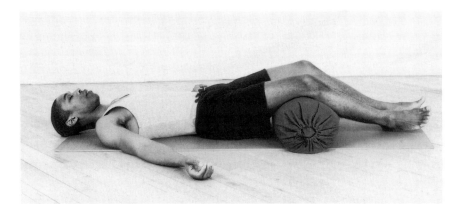

Lie flat on your back, but place the two pillows or bolster underneath your knees. This slight elevation should take pressure off your lower back and allow you to relax more deeply into the posture. As you lie there, feel the earth support your weight. Give yourself over to the rhythm of your breathing. Let yourself explore the image of being at a beach by the water's edge. In that location the sand is moist and allows your body to sink down into it. The earth holds you, nurtures you. Let your breath be like the waves, rising and falling. At the shore you cannot control the flow of the waves, so resist the temptation to interfere with your breath. Enjoy the pauses in between. Let the posture carry you to a place of tranquillity and calm. Any tension that is in you, let it be carried away by the tide . . .

VARIATIONS ON THIS *ASANA* SERIES

Before you begin your physical practice, quiet your mind with the practice of *pranayama.* Try *ujjayi pranayama* (see page 36), Alternate Nostril Breathing (see page 151), or the *Kriya* Yoga Breath (see page 153).

Pick a *kosha* upon which to direct your attention (see page 93), and focus your *asana* practice upon it.

Follow this *asana* practice with a meditation on the chakras (see page 98), to create balance among them. Meditate for a few minutes on the *mantra* (sound) and *yantra* (shape) that correspond to each of the seven chakras. Or if you prefer, pick one chakra, and focus your attention solely on its *mantra* and *yantra.*

GLOSSARY

ABHYASA: with "best effort," a clue as to how to approach one's yoga practice

AHAMKARA: the part of the mind that contains ego or the quality of I-ness (It asks "What does this have to do with me?")

AJNA: a subtle energy center located near the pituitary gland, the "point of command," the point through which divine inspiration, creativity, and karma (actions to be completed) are initiated; thoughts are quieted by focusing on this area, intuition (one's internal, or third eye) is revealed by directing one's attention to this area

AJNA BHEDANA: piercing the command center; the process of directing one's energy and awareness of mundane, temporal concerns into the third eye (one's internal, higher vision) to gaze upon the infinite nature of one's existence

AMRITA: the sweet nectar that yoga teaches is at the core of one's being

APANA: the downward moving quality of energy related to excretion and destruction

ASANA: though translated literally from the Sanskrit as "seat," *asanas* are more commonly referred to as "postures," the physical exercises one practices in hatha yoga

ASHTANGA: a style of hatha yoga that consists of six series, each one increasingly more difficult; ashtanga is learned progressively; few people in the world have advanced to the latter series

AVIDYA: the collection of habits and mental beliefs that limit one from experiencing the fullness of existence

AYURVEDA: the science, or knowledge, of life; a several-thousand-year-old scientific, holistic approach to medicine

BHARATI, SHUDDHANAND: a Tantric Master who initiated Alan and Mani Finger into yoga during the course of his visits to their home in South Africa

BRAHMANA: the feeling of expansion; the feeling of simultaneous absorption of *prana* throughout every aspect of the physical body

BUDDHI: the aspect of the mind related to intelligence, whether instinctual, rational, or enlightened

DESIKACHAR, T. K. V.: a Western-educated engineer before studying yoga with his father, Tirumalai Krishnamacharya; the highly respected Desikachar continues teaching in the tradition of his father, adjusting the practice to the individual needs of the student

DOSHA: refers to one of the three bodily humors (*Vata, Pitta, Kapha*) that bridge the mind and the body

DRISTI: gaze where one's focus is directed

FINGER, MANI: a yoga master and father of Alan Finger

HATHA YOGA: describes a set of practices designed to purify the body to prepare it for experiencing higher levels of consciousness, in particular uninterrupted bliss; it achieves this by balancing the opposing polarities within a person (*ha* means "sun," *tha* means "moon") to achieve a state of union, which is yoga

HATHA YOGA PRADIPIKA: a yoga text written in the 1300s whose focus is both the physical practices of hatha yoga as well as the meditation practices of raja yoga

IDA: one of the primary energy channels, it deals with the cooling/passive aspects of one's being

INDRIYAS: refers to the five senses: touch, taste, hearing, smell, and sight

ISHTA DEVATA: personalized deity, a Hindu concept in which one is assigned a god to look after one throughout life

ISHTA SADHANA: one's personalized daily spiritual practice

ISHTA YOGA: the system of yoga developed by Mani and Alan Finger and taught at Yoga Zone studios; the acronym ISHTA, the Integrated Science of Hatha, Tantra, and Ayurveda, is derived from the Sanskrit word *ishta*, which means "personalized"; ISHTA yoga is a style of yoga that adapts to the needs of the individual

IYENGAR, B. K. S.: the author of *Light on Yoga* and *Light on Pranayama*, two of the most popular yoga texts of the modern era; he was initiated into yoga by his brother-in-law Sri Tirumalai Krishnamacharya; his approach is very detail- and alignment-oriented

JOIS, J. P. S. PATTABHI: a student of Professor T. Krishnamacharya, he was initiated into, and now is the leading teacher of, ashtanga yoga, an athletic form of hatha yoga

KAIVALYA: space created from the Lower Mind, the world of the senses

KAPHA: one of the three humors, it refers to the combination of water and earth in the body, that which provides it with structure

KESHERTRAM: a physical point located on the outside of the body that relates to a subtle energy center located within the body

KRISHNAMACHARYA, SRI TIRUMALAI: a twentieth-century yoga teacher whose knowledge of yoga was of mythic proportion; living one hundred years (dying in 1989), he was the teacher of T. K. V. Desikachar (his son), B. K. S. Iyengar (his brother-in-law), and J. P. S. Pattabhi Jois, three teachers who have been instrumental in making yoga known to the world outside of India

KRIYA YOGA: the yoga of actions that purify one's consciousness, directing it toward spirituality

LANGHANA: the feeling of contraction or simultaneous release of all aspects of one's physical being

MANAS: perceptions

MARMA POINT: a point where consciousness and physicality diverge; directing energy into a *marma* point initiates a release of trapped energy

MAYA: the illusion that the world of the senses is all that exists

MUDRA: an energy seal

NADIS: energy pathways that sometimes mimic but are not the network of nerves in the physical body

NISHRAISANANDA, SWAMI: an influential teacher in the lives of Mani and Alan Finger, whose scientific approach to the study of yoga inspired them to approach their own teachings from a practical, nonmystical standpoint

PATANJALI: a renowned Indian scholar whose biographical details are largely unknown, but whose work, the *Yoga Sutras,* is considered by many to be the definitive compilation of yoga knowledge

PINGALA: one of the primary energy channels; it relates to the activating qualities of one's being

PITTA: one of the three bodily humors, it is the combination of fire and water and is related to all digestive functions (physical, mental, and emotional)

POWER YOGA: a derivative of ashtanga yoga, it is also often used as a catch-all term by health clubs to describe a challenging yoga class

PRAKRITI: one's constitution, set the moment the soul enters the being at conception

PRANA: life force, the energy that gives life to one's being

PRANAYAMA: exercises related to the breath in which one directs and extends the flow of life force into and out of the body

PRATYAHARA: the withdrawal of the senses away from the outside world

RAJA YOGA: the so-called "royal path," it concerns itself with the meditation practices one may employ to feel the state of oneness of yoga at one's core

SAMADHI: the state of bliss, where all disturbances in the mind field are neutralized and one experiences pure universal consciousness

SAMANA: the quality of energy related to digestion and one's internal fire

SANSKRIT: the classical language of India, a language based on sound vibration whose initial purpose was to transmit spiritual concepts; it is the original language of yoga

SHUSUMNA NADI: the central energy channel in one's being, located within the spinal cord

SIVANANDA, SWAMI: prominent twentieth-century yoga teacher instrumental in spreading the knowledge of yoga to the West

SMRITI: the quality of mind related to one's memories and past experiences

STHIRA: steadiness

SUKHA: ease

TANOTI: expansion, a root word from which *tantra* originates

TANTRA: an approach to yoga which embraces all experience as divine and inherently capable of expanding one's awareness into a state of liberation, free from the limitations of the mind and body

TAPAS: heat used for purification

TRAYATI: liberation, a root word from which *tantra* originates

UDANA: the upward moving quality of energy that relates to speech and spirituality

UJJAYI PRANAYAMA: a special type of breathing in which the area at the back of the throat is slightly constricted to slow down the intake and release of breath

VAIRAGYA: nonconcern for result

VATA: one of the three bodily humors, the combination of air and space, it is responsible for all movement in the body

VEDAS: the oldest and four of the most sacred books of Hinduism (the *Rig-Veda, Atharva-Veda, Yajur-Veda,* and *Sama-Veda*); references to yoga in these books have helped scholars trace its origins

VENKATESANANDA, SWAMI: inspirational teacher of Mani and Alan Finger from the Sivananda lineage

VIKRITI: one's condition as it relates to one's conceived constitution

VINIYOGA: a style of hatha yoga whose name is derived from its method of instruction, *vinyasa-krama,* step-by-step progressions; espoused by Sri Krishnamacharya and continued by his son T. K. V. Desikachar

VINYASA (or *vinyasa-krama*): refers to a step-by-step progression; when this concept is applied to the practice of *asana,* one allows the breath (and not the mind or body) to initiate and dictate the physical movements

VIVEKANANDA, SWAMI: a celibate yogi who introduced yoga to the United States at the World Parliament of Religions in 1893

VRTTIS: modifications or disturbances in one's mind field

VYANA: the quality of energy in one's being that relates to circulation

YOGANANDA, PARAMAHANSA: a leading spiritual figure of the twentieth century whose Self-Realization Fellowship teaches kriya yoga; initiated Mani Finger into yoga

YOGA NIDRA: this term describes the state of sleepless sleep one can enter, a state of relaxation that is in between waking and dream sleep; it can be achieved through the systematic practice of a prescribed sequence

YOGA SUTRAS: a collection of 195 Sanskrit aphorisms organized by Patanjali, an ancient Indian scholar, that are considered an authoritative source of yoga instruction

YOGI: one who practices yoga

YOGIRAJ: the title given to a yoga master

ACKNOWLEDGMENTS

Thanks to Liz Royles and Al Bingham for working with me and helping to put forty-one years of teachings into this book. I give grateful acknowledgment to the work done by Beverley Murphy in formulating and systematizing the ISHTA teachings into one of the most sophisticated teacher training programs in the world; many thanks to Jean Koerner, who has worked closely and continues to work closely with me in spreading the teachings of ISHTA yoga; and thanks to Bob Murphy for his endless support and undying faith in taking care of the business affairs relating to these teachings. Thanks go to senior teachers Kara Sekular, Rachel Zinman, Jackie Peresman, Gina Menza, Jennifer Monness, Carol Silverman, Marjorie Rosenfield, Melissa Brasier, Dave Jackson, Katrina Repka, and the entire teaching staff for their dedication and support; to senior teachers Douglass Stewart and Carrie Parker-Gastelu for their patience and poise in posing for the pictures; and to my teachers in the lineage to whom I am indebted—Paramahansa Yogananda, Swami Venkatesananda, Swami Nishraisananda, Suddhanand Bharati, and my father, Yogasvarananda Mani Finger. Also, thanks to pioneer students and teachers Lisa Bennett-Matkin and Charles Matkin, who have helped carry the flame in ISHTA and continue with commitment and passion for these teachings.

I would like to acknowledge the spiritual work done by Rod Stryker, the only initiated ISHTA student into Yogiraj. He has continued in the style of Yogananda and Venkatesananda by traveling the world and spreading the ISHTA teachings. Thank you, Rod.

Special thanks to senior teacher Donna Coogan for her endless support and effort in creating this book and in the development of ISHTA yoga.

Thanks to Michael Gordon, owner of Bumble & Bumble, who brought me to New York and graciously supported me as I got established. And to Howard Maier of Yoga Zone, who made the television show, catalogue, and a full line of videos around my teachings of ISHTA yoga.

On the publishing side, thanks to Annetta Hanna, Pam Krauss, and Laura Motta at Clarkson Potter/Three Rivers Press.

To my children, Tevya, Deva, and Sammy, for the joy they continue to provide me; to my brother, Ron, and his wife, Pat, for their unconditional love and support of me and the ISHTA teachings; to my sister, Lisa, and her husband, Selwyn, two of my earliest students and longtime admirers; and, of course, to my parents, Mani and Bex. Words cannot express my gratitude for all they have given to me. To each and everyone, *Namaste, Hari Om, Om Tat Sat.*

INDEX

ABOUT THE AUTHOR

Alan Finger, founder of Yoga Works, Yoga Zone, and Be Yoga Studios, is a second-generation Yoga Master who has been practicing yoga for more than forty years. His path began as a teenager in his native South Africa under the tutelage of his father, Kavi Yogiraj Mani Finger. From the age of fifteen, Alan has dedicated his life to an in-depth study of yogic traditions and the scientific exploration of the exact blend of postures, breathing, and meditation that accesses human potential to the fullest and benefits all levels of being. Alan became a Western Yoga Master and developed a form of yoga called ISHTA yoga, the "Integrated Science of Hatha, Tantra, and Ayurveda," a physical and spiritual form of yoga that addresses the individual needs of each student who practices it. He came to America, starting in Los Angeles, where he opened his first studio, Yoga Works, with Maty Ezrati, bringing these very pure teachings to the Western culture.

Alan's yoga is a modern, dynamic distillation of spiritual traditions blended into a form of yoga that is joyful, accessible, and vibrant. His knowledge is spiced with humor. He has a stillness that calms and an energy you can feel. At the end of each of his classes he sends his students on their way with this traditional mantra: *Hari Om, Om Tat Sat* ("Immerse yourself in unconditional love and saturate yourself in unlimited consciousness.") Alan is currently based in New York and teaching at Be Yoga. For more information, please go to www.beyoga.com.